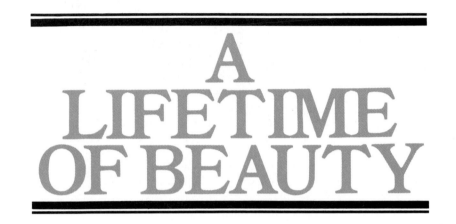

A LIFETIME OF BEAUTY

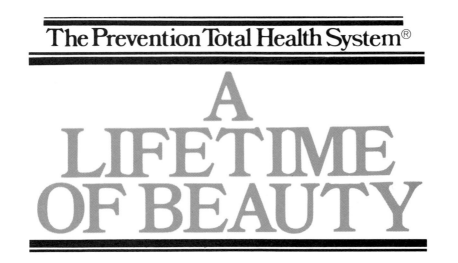

The Prevention Total Health System®

A LIFETIME OF BEAUTY

by Sharon Faelten
and the Editors of **Prevention**® Magazine

Rodale Press, Emmaus, Pennsylvania

Printed in the United States of America on recycled paper containing a high percentage of de-inked fiber.

Library of Congress Cataloging in Publication Data

Faelten, Sharon.
    A lifetime of beauty.

(The Prevention total health system)
On t.p. the circled symbol "R" is superscript following "Prevention" in the statement of responsibility and following "system" in the series.
    Bibliography: p.
    Includes index.
    1. Beauty, Personal. 2. Grooming for men.
I. Prevention (Emmaus, Pa.) II. Title. III. Series.
RA776.98.F34   1985   646.7'044
85-12640

ISBN 0-87857-553-7   hardcover
2 4 6 8 10 9 7 5 3 1   hardcover

NOTICE

This book is intended as a reference volume only, not as a medical manual or guide to self-treatment. If you suspect that you have a medical problem, we urge you to seek competent medical help. Keep in mind that nutritional and health needs vary from person to person, depending on age, sex, health status and total diet. The information here is intended to help you make informed decisions about your health, not as a substitute for any treatment that may have been prescribed by your doctor.

The Prevention Total Health System®

Series Editors: William Gottlieb, Mark Bricklin
A *Lifetime of Beauty* Editors: Sharon Faelten, Jan Bresnick, Carol Keough
Writers: Sharon Faelten (Chapters 1, 2, 3, 4, 5, 7, 9, 12), Lewis Vaughn (Chapter 6), Stefan Bechtel (Chapter 8), Leah C. Breier and Heidi Rodale (Chapter 10), Peggy Sealfon (Chapter 11)
Research Chief: Carol Baldwin
Associate Research Chief, Prevention Health Books: Susan Nastasee
Assistant Research Chief, Prevention Health Books: Holly Clemson
Researchers: Jill Polk, Carole Rapp, Martin Wood, Pamela Boyer, Kimberlee Crawford, Jan Eickmeier
Copy Editor: Jane Sherman
Copy Coordinator: Joann Williams
Art Director: Jerry O'Brien
Art Production Manager: Jane C. Knutila
Designers: Lynn Foulk, Alison Lee
Project Assistants: Lisa Gatti, Margot J. Weissman
Illustrators: Bascove, Susan Blubaugh, Susan Gray, Mary Anne Shea, Wendy Wray
Director of Photography: T. L. Gettings
Photo Editor: Margaret Skrovanek
Staff Photographers: Angelo M. Caggiano, Carl Doney, Mark Lenny, Alison Miksch, Margaret Skrovanek, Christie C. Tito
Photographic Stylists: Anne Hakanson, Renee R. Keith
Photo Researcher: Donna Lewis
Production Manager: Jacob V. Lichty
Production Coordinator: Barbara A. Herman
Composite Typesetter: Brenda J. Kline
Production Administrator: Eileen Bauder
Office Personnel: Susan K. Lagler, Roberta Mulliner

Contents

Preface

The Practical Art of Grooming

Beauty is not just in the eye of the beholder.

It is also in the eye of the beholdee.

But which is most important: to look good to others, or to *feel* good because you know you look good?

Contemporary opinion would probably favor the second choice. But I wouldn't be too quick to dismiss the importance of how our appearance strikes those around us.

I learned that lesson as a cub reporter on a big-city newspaper. I used to go to work wearing an open-neck, short-sleeve shirt, khaki pants and desert boots. In warm weather I wore short pants. I was after stories, not fashion awards. But although I did get my stories, I didn't get much in the way of recognition. One day the publisher sent around a memo saying that reporters ought to shine their shoes. Looking down at my own unpolishable suede boots and the well-shined shoes of the other reporters in the city room, I realized I had received a MESSAGE.

The next week I began wearing a white shirt and a tie, a jacket and stylish new Italian shoes that had a sheen that went beyond shine and well into the solar flare lumen level.

Now this sounds silly, but it's true. In a short time, I was promoted, promoted again, and soon became news editor. Which, I can tell you, made me feel a whole lot better than just feeling good because I looked good.

Sure, the top management people knew I was a good journalist, but professional skills are never, in real life, as persuasive as perceived personality. My appearance—although I hadn't meant it to—had been making a statement. A false statement. When I modified that statement into one that reflected what I really felt—hey, I'm a responsible person!—I began communicating.

Sending untrue messages with your appearance—without ever meaning to—can be a problem at any stage or station of life. A vigorous, active and creative person of 60 may unwittingly be saying he or she is outdated and quaint just because their appearance is. And that in turn can make people treat them like a senior citizen instead of the 40-year-old they are in mind and spirit. A warm and friendly person can come across as severe and dull if their appearance says they are. Some people will get past the false messages to know another's true character—others simply won't have the time.

There is no need to feel guilty or hesitant about grooming, be you man or woman. Nor is there any trickery or deceit to grooming, no matter how sophisticated. Our public "face" is always special. When we speak, we don't just blurt out every phase that's bouncing around in our head. Rather we choose our words with care, modulate our tone, make appropriate gestures and try to be as expressive and interesting as we can. It's the same with personal appearance. Grooming is a crucial part of communication. To ignore it is to ignore people. To improve it is to enhance all your relationships. That's why *A Lifetime of Beauty* is such an important part of The Prevention Total Health System.®

Mark Bricklin

Executive Editor, **Prevention**® Magazine

1

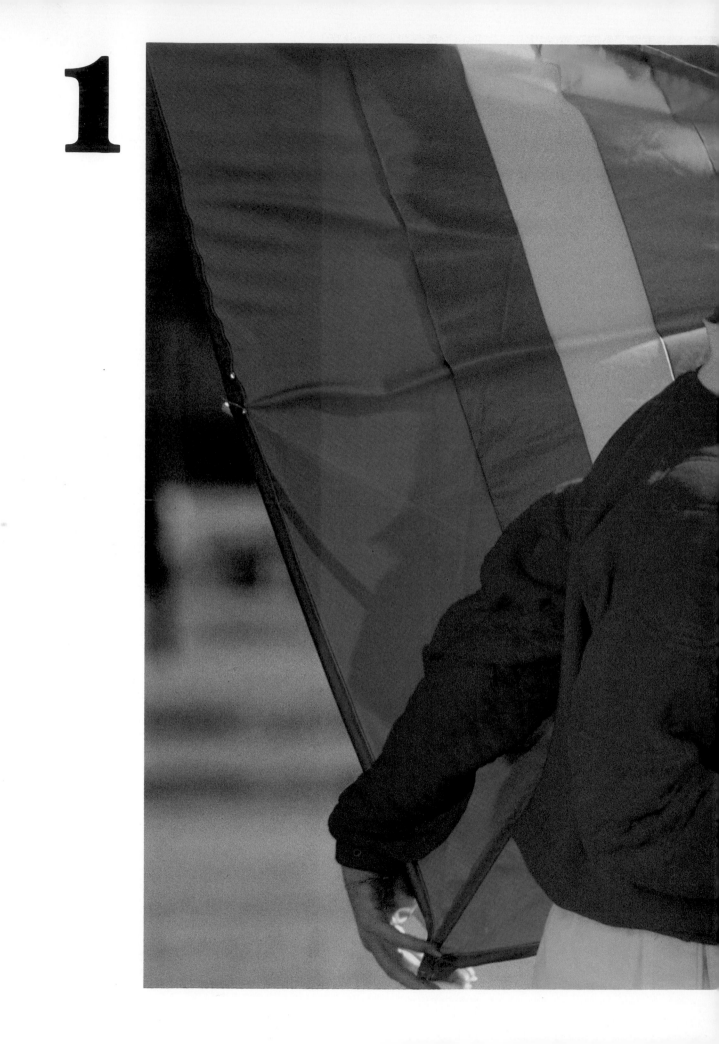

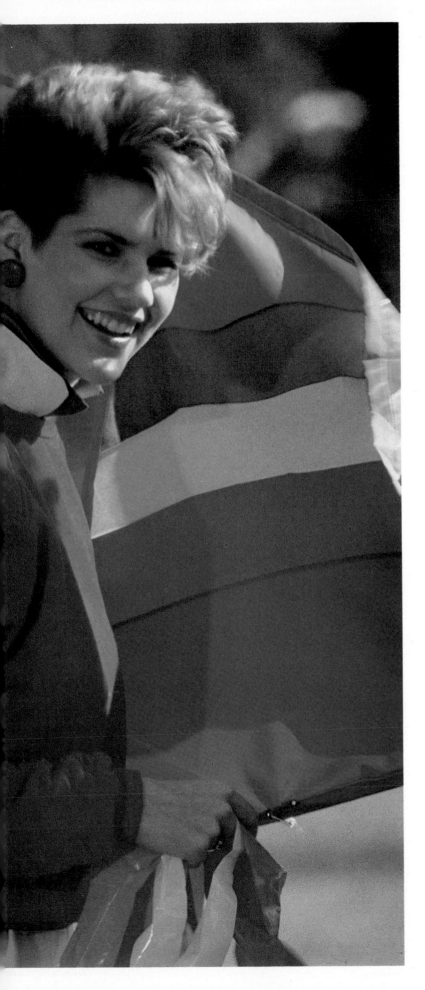

Looking Good, Feeling Good

Learning to make the most of your looks can help you to get the most out of life. It's called healthy narcissism.

Working to become more beautiful is sometimes called narcissistic—a word loaded with negative implications. Yet trying to improve your appearance is a very *healthy* thing to do. This effort does not necessarily spring from self-involvement or vanity; rather, it can be the natural result of a true respect you feel for both yourself and those around you. Furthermore, being attractive can lead to all sorts of wonderful things, ranging from an improved feeling of self-worth to (possibly) a better-paying job. Becoming more beautiful is, in fact, *healthy narcissism,* and the health benefits are physical, emotional and psychological.

Look at your mouth, for example. What makes a winning smile? Clean, pink gums that hug a full set of white, even, stain-free teeth—marks of a healthy mouth and the result of good dental hygiene.

The link between beauty and health, of course, doesn't stop at your mouth. In countless ways, skin, hair and nails that are well groomed are invariably healthier than if they had been neglected.

This concept of healthy narcissism extends to your emotional and spiritual well-being, affecting the way you interact with others and improving the quality of your life. After all, pride and self-esteem are not luxuries, but are essential to good health and happiness.

"The love you have for yourself is the nucleus of all motivation," says Perry W. Buffington, Ph.D., an Atlanta psychologist. "If you love yourself, you feel worthy. If you feel worthy, you feel competent. If you feel competent, you're ready to achieve and work and love."

How do you set off that chain reaction? By caring about yourself—a caring that can be reflected in good grooming.

"With my patients, I start with physical appearance," says Dr. Buffington. "It's probably the most important factor in people's self-esteem. I ask them what they don't like about the way they look, then let them change it for the better. Such simple modifications are the fastest routes to self-worth."

THE PSYCHOLOGY OF BEAUTY

While it would be simplistic to say you can buy happiness in a jar of cold cream, the idea isn't really so far-fetched. Certainly if the face that gazes back at you from the mirror is an attractive one, you feel happier than you would if it were homely. If your mirror is a source of depression, healthy narcissism can lead you to improve on the looks you were born with. Chances are, you'd start with makeup.

"Cosmetic products might only

Self-Adornment: The Oldest Art Form

The Cro-Magnon people did it. So did the kings and queens of Egypt. In fact, artifacts discovered in ancient historical sites prove that men and women have enhanced their appearance—often quite elaborately—in one way or another for hundreds of thousands of years. And virtually every culture in the world practices some form of self-adornment. Queen Elizabeth I, for example, owned *80* wigs to cover her bald head. In this portrait (right) she wears a ruff; it's thought she inadvertently made this style popular while just trying to conceal a long neck. In Japan, professional consorts known as geishas (center) have worn elaborate hairpins, dramatic facial makeup and other glamorous finery for hundreds of years in their roles as singers, dancers and conversationalists. The Hindu girl (far right) wears a gold nose ring anchored to her ear with a gold chain to signify that she's married.

According to anthropologists, the practice of beautifying and adorning the body seems to be universal, satisfying a need as basic and inherent as the needs for food, shelter, love and security.

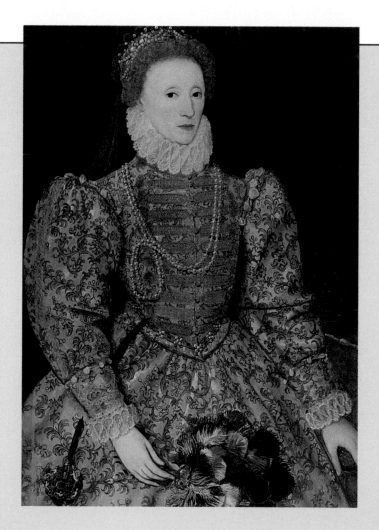

touch the skin, but their beneficial effects on the whole person are profound," say the authors of The Cosmetic Benefit Study, an analysis of the benefits of cosmetic use, including the motives and attitudes of cosmetic users, that was initiated by the Cosmetic, Toiletry and Fragrance Association. "Products such as skin and body care lotions; moisturizers; shampoos; hair conditioners; hair coloring products; eye, lip, cheek and nail products; cleansers; fragrances; and powders and deodorants help people to feel their best in almost every relationship that life has to offer . . . [satisfying] psychological needs such as security, belongingness, ego fulfillment and self-actualization. These are very human needs, and using cosmetic products to satisfy these needs is a very human thing to do," according to the study.

GREAT EXPECTATIONS

Good grooming has far-reaching effects because, like it or not, others perceive attractive people as "kind, sociable, interesting, sexually warm, poised and self-assertive," according

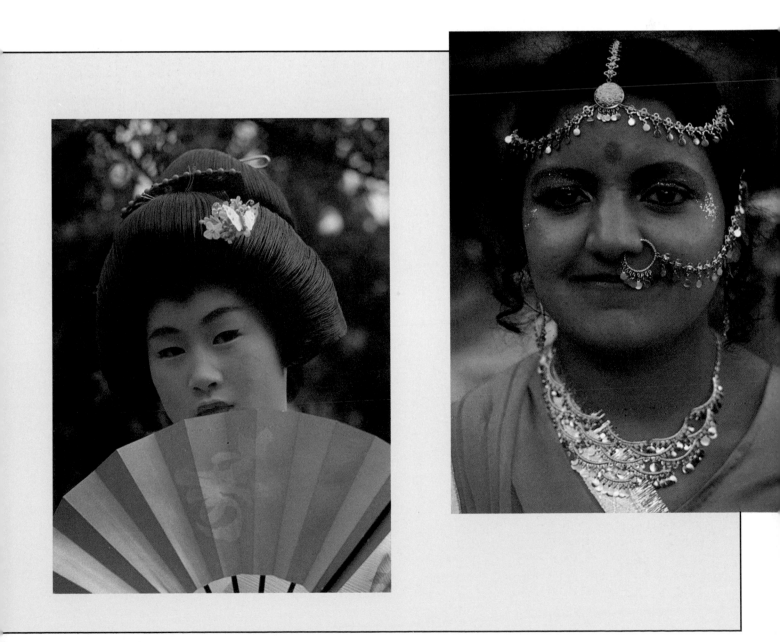

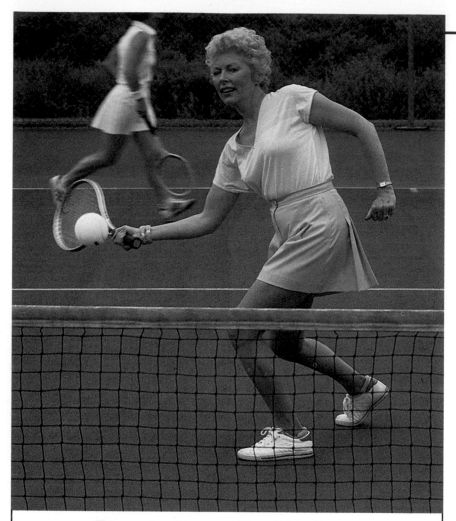

Beauty Care, Health Care

Can looking good have an effect on your health? Yes, say the experts.

Taking care of your skin provides a good example. Using a moisturizer with a built-in sunscreen not only keeps your skin smooth, delays wrinkles and prevents age spots but also can help prevent skin cancer. By the same token, wearing lipstick, because it moisturizes your lips and shields them from the harmful rays of the sun, helps prevent lip cancer while it enhances your mouth. Exercising to trim your waistline also improves the health and vitality of your heart and lungs.

In many ways, people who attempt to enhance their appearance tend to be healthier than people who aren't concerned with their looks.

to Thomas F. Cash, Ph.D., associate professor of psychology at Old Dominion University in Virginia. Unattractive people—including those who could be attractive but don't make the effort—are perceived as just the opposite. In a competitive job market, appearing well groomed can make the difference, for example, between getting or not getting a job, or getting one at a higher salary. That's the conclusion of a study conducted by Judith Waters, Ph.D., professor of psychology at Fairleigh Dickinson University in New Jersey. One hundred and twenty personnel managers and employment counselors in New York, Chicago and Los Angeles looked at either "before" or "after" photos of eight supposed job applicants, women between the ages of 25 and 55. One set of photos showed the women "as is," without makeup or any special hairstyle. The "after" photos reflected subtle changes in hair color, hairstyle and makeup— changes any woman could do herself, with know-how.

Based on the women's resumés and pictures alone, the prospective employers hired the well-groomed women at starting salaries that were 8 to 20 percent higher than those offered to the less well-groomed women. The results imply that if two people with similar experience and credentials are competing for a salary, job or promotion, the better-groomed individual will have a significant edge—especially for entry-level positions. (See pages 82-83 for an example of the sort of makeover done on the women in the study.)

It's important to note that "although people may also hold some negative attitudes about attractive people—that they are self-centered, for instance—research has shown that these negative views are typically outweighed by positive ones," says Dr. Cash.

KNOWLEDGE IS BEAUTY

The positive effects of good grooming are by no means limited to women or the young. As you'll learn in chapter 8, many men are as style-conscious as women. And older people need to pay more, not less, attention to grooming. After age 40, your skin becomes drier, your hair becomes thinner, and your perceptions about yourself change. (Facial lines that look minuscule to others seem as ominous to you as the San Andreas Fault.) You can't ignore these special changes. If anything, you need to learn more than ever about grooming.

One might say "knowledge is beauty" when it comes to grooming products and services. One of your primary goals should be to learn the basic workings of your skin, hair, teeth, nails and so forth so that you will be able to intelligently evaluate any grooming product or service. This knowledge will help you decide how to spend your grooming dollars by allowing you to differentiate realistic claims from unrealistic ones—claims, for example, that an anti-wrinkle cream can undo nature's work. (It can't.) Instead, you'll know how to avoid excessive wrinkling in the first place and disguise lines that are inevitable, saving yourself a lot of anxiety *and* money.

Health-conscious consumers also will be interested in the safety and effectiveness of cosmetics—the safest soaps for allergic skin, the best moisturizers for dry skin, the most effective sunscreens to prevent premature aging of the skin and so forth. Few cosmetic products and procedures are downright dangerous, but—like many tools—some can harm you if used improperly. For instance, bacteria can breed in mascara and infect your eyes unless the wand is handled properly. To prevent blemishes on their faces, people with acne-prone skin need to avoid using cosmetics that contain isopropyl myristate and certain other ingredients. And those who decide to have their legs "simonized" should carefully read the directions for waxing hair to avoid irritating their skin.

The issue of safety extends to clothing, too. For example, shoes that force you to walk like Richard III, not surprisingly, aren't good for your feet or your posture. Yet not all high heels are uncomfortable or hazardous. By learning exactly what features to look for when buying shoes, you can achieve both fashion and comfort.

All this brings to mind a memorable phrase from a "Saturday Night Live" sketch. An actor, impersonating a debonair Latin gentleman, says, "Personally, I would rather look good than feel good." Well, if

Winning Your Own Personal Beauty Contest

Looking your best has very real psychological, social and emotional benefits. Certainly, self-enhancement improves the way others see you and respond to you, improving your relationships with friends, family and co-workers. But more important, looking good improves your self-image (how you see yourself) and self-esteem (how you feel about yourself.) It starts a chain reaction that improves the quality of your life.

Making the most of your appearance may even help you feel smarter, more competent and more confident. One woman, after a beauty makeover with grooming products for her face, hair, skin and nails, said, "Because now I know I look good, I am beginning to feel better about me. It's amazing how out of a little outward confidence in one's appearance comes a whole new inward confidence in your intelligence."

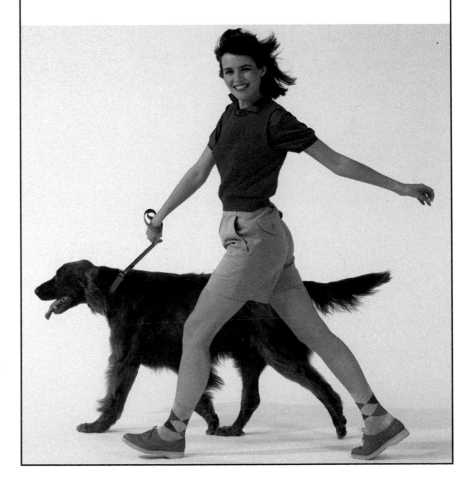

you're as smart as you are debonair, you'll realize that you can look good *and* feel good. The two are one and the same.

2

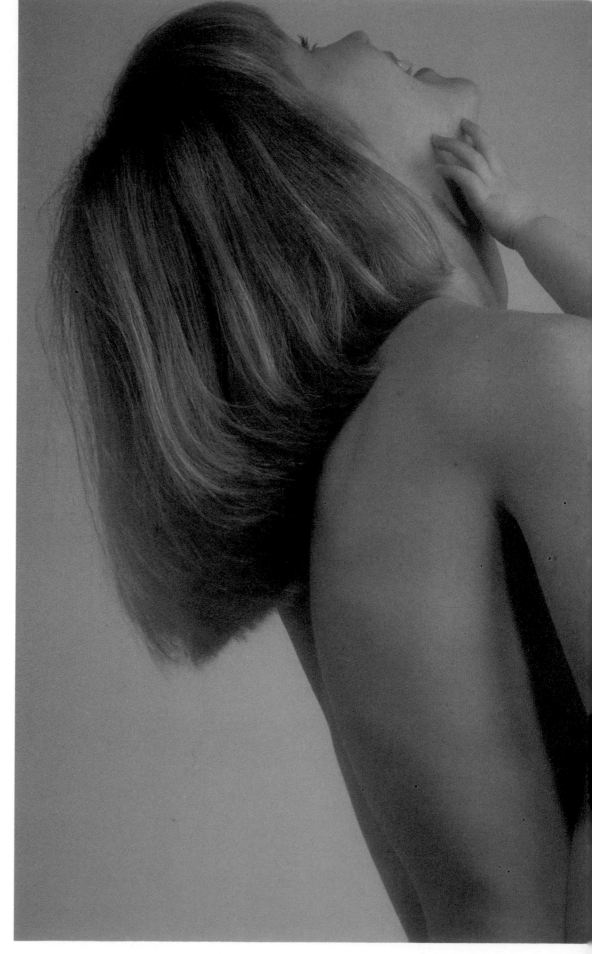

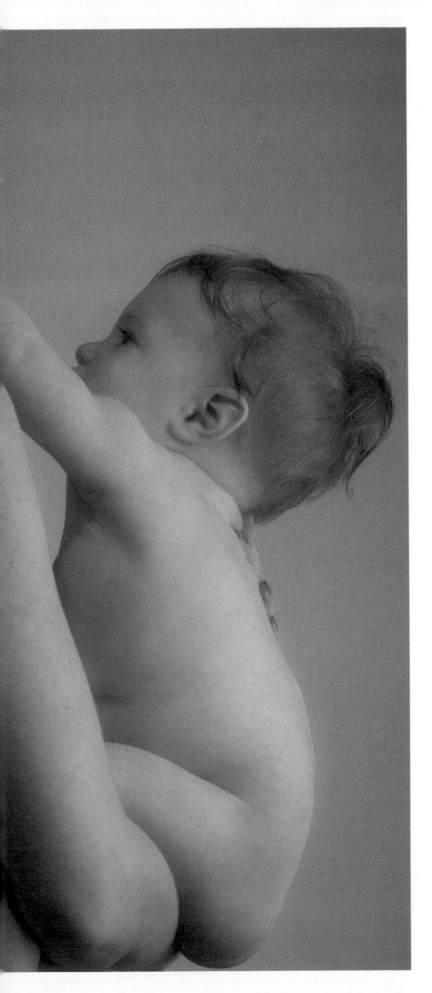

Saving Your Skin

Nature gave you a made-to-order coverall. To keep it beautiful, pamper and protect it.

Two things and two things alone can give you smooth, soft, nearly flawless skin. One is a set of parents with perfect skin; the other is a regular program of pampering and protection. You can't do much about the first condition. But conscientious care can go a long way toward transforming the skin that's so-so into a glowing head-to-toe body suit.

Just what makes skin beautiful? It's more than the absence of wrinkles, blemishes or other flaws. Truly beautiful skin exudes some special quality—its texture and tone radiate health. Fortunately, this quality is one anyone can achieve.

Protection is the first and most important step in cultivating your skin's inherent beauty. "If you lived your entire life in a closet you'd have very nice-looking skin. A very dull life. Very nice skin," quips Arnold Klein, M.D., author of *The Skin Book.*

Your skin's appearance is greatly determined by its exposure to the elements, because much of what's blamed on hormones or age is actually due to weathering—overexposure to sun, wind, chill, heat and offensive chemicals. Compare the skin on the backs of your hands with the skin on your backside or the underside of your breasts (if you're a woman). All are the same age, affected by the same hormones, yet the unexposed skin looks smoother, softer, *younger.*

But while protecting your skin will help *preserve* its natural beauty, you probably want to *enhance* you skin's natural tones and textures. You're not alone. Americans aren't skinflints— they spend about $2.6 billion a year on products that are supposed to make their skin look better: cleansing bars, moisturizers, eye creams, the whole array of bottles and jars and tubes that promise a new glow. Some of these products actually do improve your skin, while a few others may harm more than they help. You have to know the difference.

Products and protection—you have to know how to maximize both of these key elements. And the first step is to know how your skin works. Only then can you make informed, intelligent decisions about how to give your skin the best possible care.

THE SKIN YOU WERE BORN WITH

Your skin is not a passive wrapping but an active complex organ—a self-renewing coverall. It's layer upon layer of protein packed with nerve endings, with specialized cells that contain melanin (tiny granules of pigment that determine how dark your skin is) and with fibroblasts, cells that create new skin.

The very top layer of your skin—the one you can see with the naked eye—is a sheet of flat interlacing cells, called the stratum corneum, that is about as thick as the piece of paper this sentence is printed on. Washcloths and other sources of friction gradually remove these upper-most cells, while new cells migrate from the lower levels, giving you a brand new stratum corneum every 28 to 30 days.

The stratum corneum is trans-lucent, revealing the epidermis underneath, where freckles and liver spots originate.

Beneath the epidermis is the dermis, the thickest layer of all. It houses the sebaceous glands and sweat glands that percolate oil and sweat to the surface—the oil to seal in moisture and defend against fungus infection and the sweat to flush out wastes and aid in the regulation of body temperature.

The dermis is packed with collagen and elastin, proteins that make up the bulk of your skin and keep it taut, smooth and resilient. They also enable your skin to stretch when you smile and talk, then return to its original shape.

The blood vessels in the dermis deliver oxygen and other nutrients as well as the hormones or chemicals that can cause pimples or acne.

A layer of fat separates the dermis from your muscle and bone, insulating you from cold and acting as a shock absorber to protect muscles and bones from injury. It also fills out the contours of your body.

The skin structure and life cycle is much the same for newborns and children as it is for adults. So why isn't your skin as smooth and soft at 35—or 40 or 50—as it was when you were a child? Why is the skin on your elbows rougher than the skin on your face? Why do some people have very oily skin or ruddy complexions? Or acne?

As we said, heredity plays a role. If one of your parents had acne, you may have to deal with blemishes. Your ethnic background may make a difference, too. People whose ancestors originated in warm, sunny climates—the Mediterranean, Africa or equatorial South America—have generous amounts of melanin distributed evenly throughout their skin. This pigment protects the skin against overexposure to solar radiation by blocking some of the most harmful rays of the sun before they can reach the dermis and dissolve collagen and elastin. But heredity is only part of the reason your skin ages.

TIME WILL TELL

As you get older, your sebaceous glands secrete less oil, so your skin feels drier and looks parchment-paper crinkly, especially in delicate areas that get the most movement, like the eyes and neck. The stratum corneum gets a little lazy, renewing itself every 36 or 48 days instead of every 28 or 30. The dermis takes a little longer to manufacture collagen and elastin, so your skin begins to sag for lack of support. Years of exposure to sunlight can trigger concentrated explosions of melanin, known as age spots or liver spots.

Without proper care, your skin can look old at any age. As one dermatologist joked, there's only one way to reverse age: E-G-A. But although this clock has a face you can't change, time doesn't have to tell on your skin as badly as you might think. Each problem of aging that we've mentioned—and many other skin problems that are discussed later in this chapter—can be prevented, minimized or disguised. How? Obey the skin's first commandment: Thou shalt cleanse.

(continued on page 13)

Know Your Skin Type

Choosing the proper skin care regimen depends on knowing what kind of skin you have. This may not be as simple as it sounds—your skin can vary with the seasons and change with age. Still, nearly everyone's skin—whether young or not-so-young, male or female, fair or dark—falls into one of the categories we show here. Use this guide to determine which skin type most nearly matches your own.

Dry

Does your skin feel taut and drawn most of the time? Or itchy? Both are signs of dry skin.

Oily

To find out if your skin is oilier than normal, try this simple test: Before washing or showering, cut a small strip from a plain brown paper bag and rub it against your forehead 3 or 4 times. If the paper shows visible traces of oil, your skin may be oilier than normal.

Part Oily/ Part Dry

If your forehead, nose and chin—the T-zone—are oily but your cheeks aren't, you have what's known as combination skin.

Normal

If your skin is neither excessively dry nor oily in any particular areas, consider it normal.

Sensitive

If your skin is temperamental, you'll know it. Your face tends to break out in red blotches at the least provocation—say the touch of wool next to your skin or contact with perfumes in lotions or soaps. Sensitive skin may be oily, dry or somewhere in between.

A Shopper's Guide to Soap

Sculpted into rosettes, hanging from ropes or dispensed from pumps, soaps offer dozens of ways to lather up. So what makes one soap different from another? Plenty.

First, while some have a true soap base—coconut oil, tallow or other fatty acids—others have a detergent base made from petroleum. These are often milder than true soaps. Both soaps and detergents may contain deodorants, even though both kill odor-causing bacteria to some extent.

Transparent bars contain alcohol and at least 10 percent glycerin, a humectant (to attract moisture). Transparent soaps dissolve more quickly than opaque soaps so they rinse well, eliminating residues that could irritate sensitive skin. Many soaps are heavily dyed and scented, which can make them a pleasure to use if you're not allergic to these additives.

Finally, soaps with a pH higher than 7 are alkaline; those with a pH lower than 7 are acidic. Since your skin reverts to its normal pH after washing, this property is less important than overall mildness, cleansing power and rinsability.

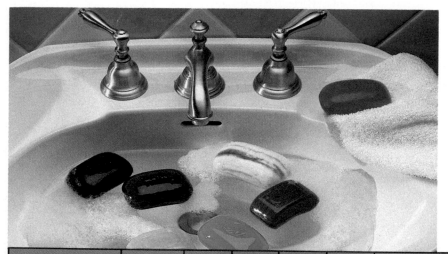

Brand	pH	Soap Base	Synthetic Base	Deodorant	Transparent	Distinguishing Characteristics
Almay Hypoallergenic Gentle Facial Soap	11.0	X				Hard-milled formula to last longer; fragrance free
Camay	10.0	X				Superfatted with coconut oil; creamy lather; good for dry skin
Caress Body Bar	7.0		X			Has a sodium cocyl isethionate base; contains bath oil; suitable for sensitive skin
Caswell-Massey English Lavender	8.0	X				Luxury French-milled soap; special packaging; perfume and color; oval shape
Clinique Soap (Mild)	n/a	X				Hard milled; superfatted; allergy tested; fragrance free
Crabtree & Evelyn Rosewater and Glycerin	n/a	X			X	Luxury transparent soap; true rose fragrance; special pink tint; oval shape
Dial	9.5-10.0	X		X		Antibacterial agents in mild, safe formula
Dove	7.0		X			Has a sodium cocyl isethionate base; mildest tested; all-purpose cleanser, particularly for dry and extra-sensitive skin

Brand	pH	Soap Base	Synthetic Base	Deodorant	Transparent	Distinguishing Characteristics
Estée Lauder Basic Cleansing Bar (Normal to Dry)	6.5		X			Nonsoap cleansing bar; has an isethionate base for mildness; contains added oils; has own carrying case; superfatted
iNatural Nutty Bar	10.5	X				Contains honey and almond meal for scrubbing; formulated for oily skin
Irish Spring	n/a	X		X		Varigated green stripes; potent fragrance
Ivory	10.5	X				Floats; efficient degreaser; all-purpose true soap
Jergens Aloe & Lanolin Soap	n/a	X				Mild; hard-milled bar soap
Johnson's Baby Bar	7.0		X			Has a mild isethionate formula appropriate for adults with sensitive skin; familiar baby-powder fragrance
Lily of Desert Beauty Bar	5.5		X			Nonalkaline; wheat flour base; aloe vera for moisturizing
Liqua 4	6.5		X			Liquid in unique soap-bar-shaped squeeze dispenser; contains moisturizers and conditioner; formulated as mild cleanser
Max Factor Gentle Cleansing Bar	n/a	X				Hard milled; formulated for normal to oily skin; has own soap dish; fragrance free
Neutrogena (original)	8.8	X			X	Superfatted transparent soap with above-average rinsing properties; proved extra mild in tests; hypoallergenic
Maja	9.0–10.0	X				Luxury castile soap (olive oil); exotic packaging and perfume
Pears	7.0+	X			X	Transparent true soap with longer-lasting formula originated in England in 1789; unique cedar and thyme scent
Purpose	10.0	X				Translucent true soap; formulated to rinse clean; mild for sensitive skin
Redken Balanced Cleansing Bar	5.0–6.0		X			Has an isethionate base; mild for sensitive skin and also formulated for normal to oily skin; has own soap dish
Safeguard	10.5		X	X		Superfatted; substantial lathering; all-purpose mild soap for all skin types; faint floral fruit and woody scent
Softsoap Brand Liquid Soap	6.5		X			Liquid cleanser; convenient and neat for quick use in kitchen, office
Tone	9.5–10.0	X				Contains glycerin and cocoa butter; yellow color; light fragrance
Weleda Rosemary Soap	8.5	X				Hard milled; made with natural plant oils; free of animal fats; pungent herbal fragrance; superfatted
Yardley English Lavender Soap	n/a	X				Hard milled; since 1770; true lavender fragrance

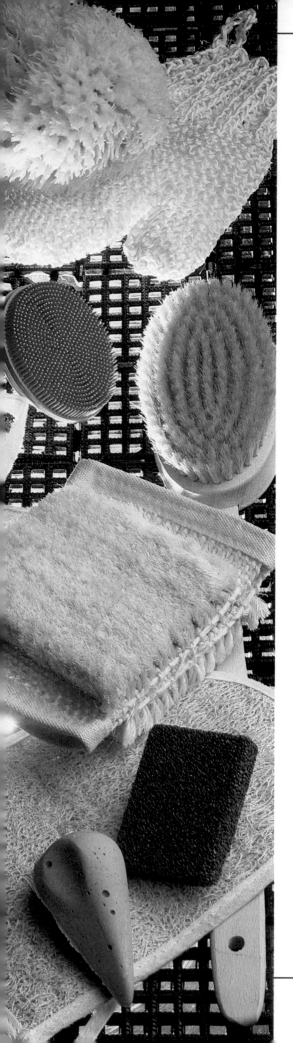

Buffing Tools to Polish Your Skin

Extra scrubbing action with the right tool can give your skin a fresh glow by buffing away dead skin cells that cling to its surface. Heels, elbows and backs, for instance, may need more polishing than you can achieve with a washcloth. Gentle scrubbing is the key to success. Follow the manufacturer's directions to avoid overdoing it.

Scrubbing Cleansers. Soaps and lotions containing fine grains of pulverized shells or other granular material can buff away stagnant surface cells along with dirt. To acclimate your skin to the increased friction, dilute the scrub with extra water. Work up to full strength gradually. Don't use scrubbing grains around your eyes.

Polyester Facial Sponges. These round or tear-drop-shaped sponges are easy to handle, durable and hygienic—they don't develop a sour smell or foster bacteria the way rubber or cellulose sponges sometimes do when left to dry. Use a mild soap along with the sponge, and rinse it thoroughly after each use. Many dermatologists feel that scrubbing with a facial sponge controls blackheads.

Sea Sponges. These porous, absorbent skeletons of marine animals have been used as body scrubbers for centuries. Two drawbacks: They tend to deteriorate and lose their abrasiveness with use and they can harbor bacteria.

Loofah Brushes and Sisal Mitts. A loofah is either the fibrous skeleton of the loofah fruit or a synthetic version. Sisal mitts are woven from a hemplike fiber. Both loofahs and sisals are strictly for below-the-neck scrubbing—they're too abrasive for the face. Loofahs and sisals are also less flexible and harder to keep clean than are polyester sponges.

Bath Brushes. Scrubbing with an ordinary bath brush is an invigorating way to slough off dead skin cells. Go easy: If the bristles curl up against your skin, you're probably pressing too hard.

Pumice Stones. Pumice is a lightweight, porous volcanic stone that's used to polish and smooth skin. It's best reserved for use on the heels, the balls of the feet and other thickly calloused spots.

Electric Brushes. These battery-operated, waterproof, circular spinning brushes often have pumice attachments for super polishing power. Because it's easier to overscrub and irritate your skin with a machine, use electric brushes only on heels or other tough areas.

MAKE A SPLASH

Cleansing the skin is like preparing a wall for a fresh coat of paint: no matter how pretty the color, the paint job will look slipshod if there are dirt and rough spots underneath. Poorly cleansed skin will look dull and flaky. The oil glands can clog and form whiteheads or pimples, even in people with dry skin. And no amount of even the finest makeup can cover these flaws.

Water alone won't cut through the thin, sticky buildup of oil, dirt, perspiration and dead skin cells, because water and oil repel each other. So you have to apply friction to loosen sticky grime and use some kind of soap or detergent (synthetic soap). (See "A Shopper's Guide to Soap" on pages 10-11.)

The type of skin you have dictates what type of soap or cleanser is best for you.

Dry or Dry/Normal Skin. With little natural oil to spare, dry or partly dry skin fares well when washed with superfatted soaps, such as Basis or Nivea, or *washable* cleansing creams. Mature skin, in particular, needs a gentle, nondrying cleanser that can be thoroughly rinsed away. Otherwise a residue of soap or irritating ingredients can further dry the skin. Be careful not to overcleanse; twice a day is usually enough.

Oily Skin. If your skin is extremely oily, wash with a strong degreaser, such as Ivory, or a nongreasy, milky cleanser that leaves no sticky film behind. If your skin is mildly oily, washing thoroughly twice a day should be adequate.

Sensitive Skin. If you have skin that breaks out easily, chances are that not just any soap will do. You're least apt to rile your skin if you wash with a mild soap such as Dove, Caress or Johnson's Baby Bar. Look for cleansers containing sodium isethionate, one of the least drying or irritating ingredients in soaps. Avoid fragrances and other superfluous additives. Sensitive skin may also be dry, so don't wash more than necessary.

Normal Skin. If you've used a variety of soaps or cleansers over the years and have never broken out in a rash or felt other discomfort, you probably have normal skin and can wash twice a day with almost any soap or cleanser that appeals to you.

Many cleansing creams—whether solids or thick lotions—do not always remove dirt thoroughly and can leave behind a sticky film, requiring a strong solvent to remove them. You're better off using a soap or cleanser that rinses off easily with plain water.

Forget anything you may have heard about soap destroying the skin's acid mantle (a thin film of oil, sweat and other secretions that covers the topmost layers of skin and defends it against bacteria). Because most soap is alkaline (with a pH of 7 to 11) and skin is mildly acidic (with a pH of 6 or 7), the majority of dermatologists believed that soaps destroyed the acid mantle and harmed the skin. Now doctors believe that pH is a minor consideration. Mildness and rinsability are more important qualities. (See "A Shopper's Guide to Soap" on pages 10-11.)

Whatever soap you choose, work up a lather in your hands or use a washcloth or sloughing pad (see "Buffing Tools to Polish Your Skin"), then spread the lather on moistened skin. Rinse thoroughly.

TONICS: THE FINAL STEP

After you've washed your face, dab your skin with a cotton ball soaked in a tonic lotion designed for your skin type. This removes the dull film left by minerals in tap water and wipes away the last traces of dirt, soap, cleanser and superfluous oil from surface cells. Here's a survey of various tonics.

Astringents. These contain a high percentage of alum, alcohol or witch hazel, which dry the skin and remove excess oil. Astringents that contain alum cause tissues around pores to swell, leaving the impression that the pores shrink.

You can use an astringent once a week or so if you have normal skin or more often if you have oily skin. Astringents are unnecessary and possibly harmful if you have dry or sensitive skin.

Toners and Fresheners. These contain a large proportion of water to remove final traces of soap and hydrate the face, and an acid to break down the residue of cleansing creams. You can make a simple toner by diluting 1 tablespoon of lemon juice or white vinegar in 2 cups of water. Or dilute Sea Breeze antiseptic lotion or witch hazel in water, one part to three. Make a fresh batch each day to prevent bacterial growth.

Clarifying Lotions. Sometimes called exfoliating lotions, clarifying lotions contain ingredients such as benzoic acid or salicylic acid that make your face look fresh and rosy by dissolving dry, dead cells from the skin's surface. Choose a product designed for your skin: a mild one for normal skin, a stronger one for oily skin.

POLISHING YOUR SKIN

Washing helps your skin's natural process of cell renewal, the continuous process of shedding old skin cells at the surface as new skin cells form and migrate upward from the epidermis below. Cell renewal occurs in a remarkably uniform pattern: for every cell layer lost at the surface, a new layer is generated below.

In your teens and twenties, cells renew themselves at a fast clip—about one layer per day. With age, cell renewal slows down gradually, so the older you get, the more time surface cells are exposed to weather, pollution and other assaults. Also, cells reaching the surface sooner are plumper than cells that take twice as long to get there—they have less time to flatten out and accumulate keratin, a tough epidermal protein. Plumper cells reflect light more uniformly, so your skin looks smoother.

Rubbing vigorously with the nubby side of a washcloth, mitt, sponge, loofah or other abrasive material aids a process called exfoliation, the removal of dead surface cells. (See "Buffing Tools to Polish Your Skin" on page 12.) Done properly, this can stimulate the birth of new cells, which may speed up cell renewal by 30 percent.

Polished this way, skin takes on the plumper, smoother, rosier characteristics of younger skin—characteristics that shine through even under makeup.

CHOOSING THE RIGHT MASK

Nearly every cosmetic company sells a facial mask, a mixture you spread on your face, allow to dry, then peel or rinse off. Masks remove dead skin cells and debris from pores, drying and temporarily tightening your skin in the process and making wrinkles less noticeable for a couple of hours. Your skin will glow slightly because masks stimulate the blood vessels to dilate. No matter what a manufacturer claims, however, a mask cannot nourish your skin. So while mask ingredients such as yogurt, avocado or honey may have cleansing properties, they won't feed your skin. Honey can even irritate your skin.

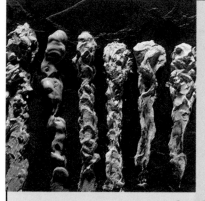

The Dirt on Clay

Betonite, silica, Fuller's earth and kaolin—the standard ingredients in clay masks—draw out impurities from the skin, pull off debris and leave your skin soft and rosy. Although clay tends to absorb oils, it acts as a temporary watertight shield to retain moisture. However, after removing the mask you should use a moisturizer, especially if your skin is dry.

Here's a guide to help you choose the clay best suited to your skin. In general, the darker the clay, the more absorbent it is.

Dark Brown. Rich in iron, for oily skin.

Green. Good for oily or part oily/part normal skin.

Rose. Delicate. Suitable for all skin types.

White. Very gentle, for very dry or sensitive skin.

People who have oily skin probably benefit most from masks—especially clay and mud masks that draw oil and impurities from the skin. Dry skin may need a moisturizing mask—usually a gel that retards moisture evaporation. A person whose skin is partly oily and partly dry may need a different mask for each area of the face—a drying mask for the forehead, nose and chin and a moisturizing mask for the rest of the face. People with normal skin can alternate between drying masks and moisturizing masks.

To apply a mask, begin with absolutely clean hands and face. Steam your face for 5 minutes, then apply the mask according to the package directions, avoiding the eye area. Once it has dried, either peel it off or rinse it off with a washcloth and some cool water.

You can make a simple, effective mask at home. Egg white makes a good tightening mask for any skin type, Add 2 tablespoons of lemon juice to the whites of two eggs, then whip with electric beaters until peaks form. Spread it on your face. Peel it off 20 minutes later, then rinse.

WATER CONSERVATION

The minute you step out of your tub or shower, reach for a moisturizing lotion and apply it. Do the same right after washing your face or hands. The moisturizer provides an oily barrier that seals in the moisture you absorb while you bathe.

Moisture is your skin's most valuable commodity, keeping it soft, supple and less prone to redness and irritation. Without enough water, the topmost layer of the skin soon can become rough, cracked, scaly and itchy.

Water makes skin more soft and elastic, explains Gary Grove, Ph.D., director of the Skin Study Center in Philadelphia. He also points out that the stratum corneum itself serves as a barrier to seal in moisture. But if you disrupt the stratum corneum—say, by washing—the barrier is disrupted and excessive water loss occurs. To prevent excessive water loss, apply an oily barrier—a moisturizing lotion.

What Makes a Moisturizer?

All moisturizers are basically a blend of oils (emollients) and water, with small amounts of helper ingredients. Here's the role each ingredient plays.

Emollients. Lanolin, lanolin alcohol, mineral oil, cocoa butter, petrolatum, isopropyl myristate and dimethicone are forms of oil that lubricate, seal in moisture and make your skin feel softer and smoother.

Emulsifiers. Glyceryl stearate, alkyl sulfates and similar substances bind ingredients so they're easy to apply and don't separate.

Humectants. Glycerin, urea, lactic acid and propylene glycol hold moisture, making the moisturizer more available to your skin.

Plant Extracts. Aloe vera, jojoba and other extracts may be added for their soothing, healing properties.

Preservatives and Stabilizers. Paraben compounds such as methylparabens and propylparabens are the most common. They prevent products from turning rancid and contaminating your skin.

Thickeners. Carbomer compounds, such as carbomer-941, blend ingredients into a uniform consistency.

Water. Water dilutes emollients, helps the product spread and hydrates the skin.

Dyes and Fragrances. Coal tar dyes, like FD&C Red No. 4, and scents make a product more attractive but can irritate sensitive skin.

People with oily or very oily skin have a built-in moisturizing system: their oil glands. So they need to moisturize only areas that are dry. Otherwise, putting oil on top of oil can smother your oil glands, promoting blackheads.

Also, many people find that an all-purpose cream or lotion may be fine for their hands and bodies, but they need a nongreasy, lighter-textured lotion for their faces. When in doubt, choose a lotion over a cream to avoid *over*moisturizing your face and clogging pores.

Certain situations dramatically increase the need for a moisturizer. Anything that disrupts the stratum corneum—sunburn or detergents,

Add Pizzazz to Your Bath

A relaxing soak in a warm bath at the end of a taxing day can be one of life's more pleasurable rituals. With a little imagination and a few simple ingredients, you can turn a tub of warm water into a sensual soak. Now, light a candle, place a little sachet nearby and add one of these to your bath:

Vinegar. Add ½ cup of white vinegar to a few inches of warm (not hot) bath water. The slightly acidic solution helps to rinse away soap residue that, left behind, could irritate sensitive skin. Vinegared bath water also counteracts vaginal infections—the organisms cannot survive in an acidic environment.

Bath Salts and Crystals. If you bathe in hard water, add ½ cup of table salt, baking soda, bath salts or bath crystals to your tub water. It helps make the water soft.

Bath Oil. If you have dry, itchy skin, especially during the winter months, add a few drops of baby oil, olive oil or commercial bath oil to your bath water after you've soaked for 10 to 15 minutes. (If you do it sooner, the oil will block out moisture instead of sealing it in.) Oil makes the tub slippery, so sit on a mat and be careful when getting out of the tub.

Colloidal Oatmeal or Cornstarch. Colloidal oatmeal (available at drugstores) and ordinary cornstarch remain suspended in bath water, gently soothing skin that may be irritated by rashes, sunburn or allergies.

Bubble Bath. A few years ago, bubble baths were blamed for infections of the urinary tract. The problem was apparently triggered in young girls who added far more bubble bath to their tub water than the directions called for and whose parents let them play in the tub for an hour or so. Used correctly—by adding only the amount specified on the label and soaking for 20 minutes or so—bubble bath is safe, according to the FDA. However, bath beads and gels contain detergents such as sodium lauryl sulfate, which strip away the skin's natural oils. They can dry and sometimes irritate the skin as well. People with dry skin would be better off using a bath oil instead of bubble bath, and people with normal or oily skin should reserve bubble baths for hot, humid months, when skin dehydration is less of a problem. To further minimize dryness, swish the suds around before you step into a bubble bath to be sure the grains are completely dissolved and as dilute as they should be.

for example—speeds up water loss. Wind speeds up evaporation, too. So activities such as bicycling, gardening, sailing and jogging call for extra protection.

Whenever you spend a day in water, body surfing, snorkeling or falling off a sailboard 20 times, your skin needs help conserving moisture. Repeated wetting and drying of the skin dissolves the cement that holds the stratum corneum together, making that layer less able to hold water. Dunking your bare hands in and out of household detergents can have the same effect.

Your skin will tell you when it needs a moisturizer. If you go without lotion for a day, your skin will probably begin to feel taut, as if it were shrinking. Don't ignore that cry for help.

ANATOMY OF A WRINKLE

A wrinkle is a crease in the skin caused by a thinning of the collagen, or supporting tissue, of the epidermis.

Some moisturizers claim to remove wrinkles and other signs of aging skin. Marketed as antiaging creams, rejuvenation formulas or cellular renewal creams, these souped-up moisturizers have a minuscule effect on wrinkles and aren't worth the extra cost. All they really do is moisturize the skin and plump out dry lines, which an ordinary moisturizer can do just as well. Dry skin doesn't cause wrinkles—but it does make them more noticeable.

Collagen is a commonly used wrinkle fighter. Collagen from animal protein makes a fairly good moisturizer, but your skin cannot absorb collagen that's applied topically—the molecules are simply too large. Nor can topically applied collagen magically stimulate your skin to produce collagen of its own. (Collagen does eliminate wrinkles for about two years when injected under the skin. See "Alternatives to Surgery" on page 150.)

Few substances, in fact, penetrate beyond the stratum corneum to the epidermis, where they could do some good. You wouldn't even want them to, because that would mean the oils and other ingredients in these products would end up floating around in your bloodstream. Other ingredients besides collagen that have not been proven to rejuvenate skin or erase wrinkles are the cellular blueprint material, RNA and DNA; superoxide dismutase, an enzyme; and vitamin E.

Moisturizers containing retinoic acid, a synthetic form of vitamin A, are the closest thing to a wrinkle eraser and may be available over the counter in a few years. Applied to the skin surface, retinoic acid increases blood flow and stimulates skin cells called fibroblasts to produce new collagen. This can help to eliminate tiny wrinkles and make deep wrinkles less noticeable. Retinoic acid also speeds up the rate of cell renewal, helping skin look younger. For now, retinoic acid is available only by prescription and is used primarily to treat acne. (Regular vitamin A has no effect on wrinkles, whether it's taken orally or applied directly to the skin.)

Since nothing you can buy in a jar can remove wrinkles, the next best course is to prevent them—or prevent any you have now from getting worse. You can start by making it a habit always to wear dark glasses in bright light, so you don't squint. Muscle actions like squinting, smiling and frowning accentuate wrinkles, deepening creases in the natural foldlines of the skin. No one recommends you give up smiling, but you could forgo frowning with no great inconvenience. And if you habitually purse your lips or grimace while deep in thought, try to break the habit.

By all means, don't do facial exercises or twist your face intentionally. Facial exercises promote wrinkling and are the worst thing you can do to your skin, according to Albert M. Kligman, M.D., director of the Aging Skin Clinic of the Hospital of the University of Pennsylvania. "The muscles of your face have one purpose only—to open and close your mouth and eyelids," says Dr. Kligman. "So your face already gets plenty of exercise."

What's more, facial muscles don't increase in size the way biceps do, so you can't build up facial muscles to take up the slack in sagging skin.

Squinting also may contribute to wrinkles, but this habit is minor league compared to the major cause of wrinkles: the sun. The sun's ultraviolet rays penetrate the stratum corneum to the epidermis, where they slowly eat away at collagen, the very same protein that antiwrinkle creams try to replace. With prolonged sun exposure, the skin develops a network of lines and wrinkles.

Wrinkles aren't the only undesirable products of solar radiation: The circular patches of light brown pigment called liver spots or age spots begin to appear at age 30 or 40. At that point, only two methods (both procedures done in a doctor's office) will remove the spots: A chemical peel (a mild acid is applied with a cotton swab to each patch of pigment) or dermabrasion (the skin is numbed, then rubbed with metal or other abrasive material). Both procedures are effective and leave no scars, but they're unpleasant and somewhat risky.

Bleaching creams, sold at drugstores, may lighten age spots slightly but won't remove them.

Wrinkles and age spots can begin to show up well before middle age, so it's never too soon to start thinking about prevention, even if you're young and your skin looks flawless.

"Few people have perfectly normal skin," says Dr. Kligman. "If you're over 30 and have been out in the sun at all, your skin shows telltale signs."

A NEW BREED OF SUNSCREENS

Some people have no choice but to spend long hours in the sun—land surveyors, sailors and outdoor sports enthusiasts, for example. But let's face it—many people go outdoors with the sole intent of soaking up as much solar radiation as possible.

Back in the 1940s sunworshipers in Miami Beach discovered that skin slathered with baby oil looked sexier, tanned faster and faded more slowly than dry-roasted skin. Manufacturers packaged oil in bronze-colored bottles, added fragrance and christened the stuff with exotic brand names—thus tanning oil was born.

Bronzed beachophiles every-where were happy as clams until unsettling reports begin to circulate around paradise that the healthy tan wasn't so healthy after all. Aside from a painful sunburn or some unsightly peeling, overexposure to the sun was proved to be the primary source of skin cancer: Radiation scrambles cellular blueprints and the result is new, diseased—and rapidly multiplying—cells.

Still, many people remained blasé or skeptical, no matter how scientific the evidence was. Soaking in the sun's warmth and energy, the prospect of cancer seemed remote to many—especially if they had jetted down to Aruba for a midwinter fix of fun and sun. Besides, many people felt they looked better—leaner, sexier, *richer*—with a tan. The appeal was hard to resist.

Then the second wave of unsettling news hit the beach: Tanning year after year alters your skin's structure, ultimately turning it into beat-up leather. Collagen dissolves, elastin disappears and skin cells toughen and harden. This time, people began to sit up on their chaise lounges and take notice. But they didn't exactly retreat to the cabana.

By and by, suntan oil manufacturers discovered that with added compounds such as para-aminobenzoic acid (PABA, a B vitamin derivative), lotions could block out or absorb the harmful rays of the sun, prolonging the amount of time people could safely spend tanning. The potential amount of protection is measured in SPFs, or Sun Protection Factors, a multiple of the amount of sun you would absorb if you weren't wearing the lotion. Wearing a sunscreen with an SPF of 8, for example, you could spend up to 8 times as much time in the sun without multiplying your exposure. If you spend 2 hours playing golf or volleyball, you would absorb only about 15 minutes' worth of sun. (Sunscreens don't block out *all* the sun—only a sunblock, such as zinc oxide or lotions with an SPF of 15 or higher, can do that. Even when you wear a sunblock, 10 to 40 percent of the light gets through—enough to burn your skin if you stay out long enough or if you have porcelain-complexioned skin with little natural melanin to protect you.)

WHY YOU SHOULD BAN TANS

Can you tan safely, as some people insist? We wish that were true. Granted, a gradually acquired tan is less damaging than an outright burn or a quick, three-day souvenir tan. But the bare fact is that all tans or burns damage the skin.

"A tan or a burn is a response to injury," says John Parrish, M.D., of Massachusetts General Hospital in Boston. "You cannot have a tan without injury. Period."

In fact, some products that "help" you tan only help you hurt yourself. Avoid tanning aids that contain 5-methoxypsoralen, which induce a tan by stimulating production of melanin in the presence of sunlight. Sold in Europe but not the United States, these photosensitizing products claim to help fair-skinned people tan instead of burn. However, the chemical is suspected of causing cancer.

Pretanning products containing the amino acid tyrosine also claim to enhance tanning. But even though they seem to be safe, they simply don't work.

And don't bother sitting in a tanning booth or other artificial tanning device to prime your skin for a midwinter vacation—or to prolong a souvenir tan. This will *not* give you a safer tan or prevent sunburn. In fact, artificial tanning may be more dangerous than the real thing: The light is as intense as the sun at high noon, or even stronger. That's exactly the time of day you should stay out of the sun. And, just like the sun, the artificially generated rays penetrate deeply, helping to cause itching, rashes, sunburn, wrinkles, premature aging and skin cancer.

"If you go out into the sun after using a tanning booth or tanning bed, the damage to your skin is even worse than using either the sun or the booth by itself," says one skin specialist.

If all this doesn't dissuade you and you elect to tan anyway, Dr. Kligman emphasizes that it's just as important to apply a sunscreen after you have a tan as before. Melanin provides only partial protection from sun-caused damage.

You're never too old to start using a sunscreen, and the closer to SPF 15 (sunblock) the better. (SPFs higher than 15 offer no significant advantage.)

"Even people over age 70 should use a sunscreen," says Dr. Kligman. "As soon as they discontinue sun exposure, the skin will recover to some degree."

Sunscreens also save the day for people who are allergic to the sun. Those who are susceptible (and anyone can develop this sensitivity) can break out in a nasty rash, swelling and what looks like sunburn if they take certain medications, use certain cosmetics or soaps with perfumes or eat certain foods that can cut sun tolerance by up to 90 percent. The list of photosensitizing substances includes:

- Hexachlorophene and essences of lemon and lime (used in some bath soaps and lotions)
- Oil of bergamot (a fragrance found in some perfumes and cosmetics)
- Saccharin (an artificial sweetener found in soft drinks and some diet snack foods)

(continued on page 22)

A Rain-or-Shine Tan?

Bronzing gels and quick-tanning lotions appeal to people who feel naked without a tan yet want to avoid sun-induced skin damage.

While both products have come a long way since their introduction 25 years ago, both take considerable skill and practice to produce anything remotely resembling a tan. In fact, you could end up looking ridiculous.

Bronzing lotions that contain iron pigments or other brown dyes are basically makeup, so they wash off with perspiration. And unless applied very evenly, they will streak. Some leave skin looking varnished.

Quick-tanning lotions that contain the colorless chemical dihydroxy acetone (DHA) react with skin protein to produce the appearance of a tan within 3 to 5 hours, without exposure to sunlight. The effect wears off in about 3 days. While the FDA considers DHA safe, you can easily end up with an uneven or unconvincing veneer: DHA reacts more readily with thicker skin on the palms or elbows, and not at all with scar tissue.

Sun Sense

Your skin converts sunshine into vitamin D to build strong bones and shiny white teeth. Spend more than a few minutes a day in its bright light, though, and those energizing rays seep into your epidermis to dissolve collagen and elastin, the proteins responsible for firm, smooth skin. But you can worship the sun and reap its benefits—physical and psychological—without sacrificing your future good looks. Here's how.

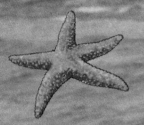

If you are fair skinned and have blue, green or hazel eyes and light hair, chances are you will burn more easily and suffer more long-lasting damage than people with darker skin, eyes and hair. You should use a sunscreen with an SPF of no less than 15. Apply lotion at least 45 minutes before you expect to go outdoors, to give your skin plenty of time to absorb the protective ingredients. Reapply liberally and often.

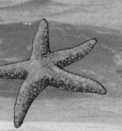

Pay special attention to your nose, lips, shoulders and other easy targets. Also, skin that's rarely exposed to the sun, such as the upper thighs and torso, are more likely to burn than previously tanned areas.

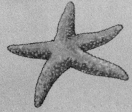

Trees, umbrellas and patio awnings cut sun exposure by only half, so you can't assume you're safe in the shade. For added protection, wear a straw hat or visor and long-sleeved, light-colored clothing. White, khaki, beige and pastels reflect more light away from your skin than dark colors.

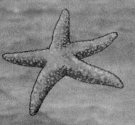

Ultraviolet light zips right through water to your skin. And when you're battling sun, wind *and* water, nothing succeeds like excess: Apply a sunscreen liberally before you go in the water.

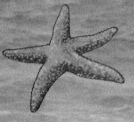

Skiers, take note: At higher elevations, the atmosphere is thinner and more ultraviolet light reaches you. Also, snow reflects the sunlight reaching the ground, increasing the amount to which you're exposed.

Acne-prone people use sunlight to help clear up their blemishes. However, if you're taking retinoic acid (Accutane) or tetracycline (an antibiotic sometimes prescribed for acne), your skin may be unusually sensitive to sunlight. If you take either of these drugs, you may want to stay out of the sun.

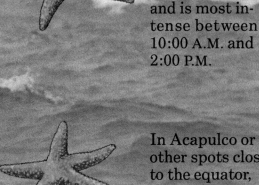

Take a long lunch hour from tanning. The sun is highest in the sky and is most intense between 10:00 A.M. and 2:00 P.M.

In Acapulco or other spots close to the equator, the sun is twice as strong as it is in Seattle or other northern locales. So your sunblock is twice as important when you're at the earth's waistband.

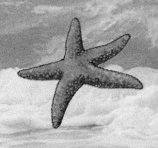

Clouds filter out only a small number of harmful rays, so don't let overcast skies tempt you to forgo your sunscreen or stay out longer.

- Celery, figs, parsnips, vanilla, lime and other citrus fruits.

Sunscreens are available to suit every complexion, says Dr. Kligman. People with oily skin should use light, greaseless, alcohol-based lotions to avoid clogging pores. And some brands of foundation makeup, discussed in chapter 5, contain sunscreens.

Sunscreens gradually lose their potency as they sit on the shelf. You may get only a fraction of the protection you think you're getting if you apply a sunscreen that's sat in the back of your bathroom closet for a few years. To be safe, use a product within three years of buying it (or before the expiration date, if one is listed).

Also, because some sunscreens absorb sunlight, they raise skin temperature and promote perspiration. So be sure to drink plenty of water or fruit juice if you're running or biking or otherwise exerting yourself. (Since citrus juice can irritate or burn your lips or the skin around your mouth when its exposed to sunlight, sip it through a straw or choose a noncitrus drink.)

DON'T DO ANYTHING RASH

Is your skin usually itchy? Blotchy? Flaky? Maybe even allergic? Always on the verge of breaking out in red blotches despite devoted efforts to keep it scrupulously clean and pampered? Then you have sensitive skin.

Sensitive skin is prone to rashes that may be triggered by simple irritation (mechanical or chemical action) or allergy (an immune reaction to ingredients that don't bother most people). Either way, treatment is the same: Track down the cause, avoid it and nurse the skin back to good health.

Dermatologists say that makeup and cosmetics are a growing cause of allergic rashes. Even hypoallergenic products can trigger a rash in some people. That doesn't necessarily mean that the manufacturer goofed. Hypoallergenic products are simply less likely to cause adverse reactions than the usual line of cosmetics. Because anyone can be allergic to anything, no product can be guaranteed 100 percent free of allergens.

A spokesperson for the U.S. Food and Drug Administration (FDA) says that no official standard exists for hypoallergenic products. The cosmetic industry sets its own criteria. Because fragrances are the single most common cause of cosmetic allergies, scents are usually the first item to be omitted in anything marketed as hypoallergenic. For many

---

Beauty Marks You Can Do Without

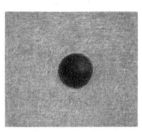

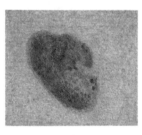

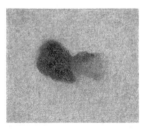

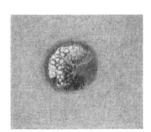

Marilyn Monroe had a mole, euphemistically called a beauty mark. So do plenty of other people. Some moles look cute or sexy; others are simply a nuisance. But no matter what you think of them, these patches or knobs of dark pigment should be watched carefully. Moles are the sort of disorganized tissue that can develop into cancer, especially if you have a history of skin cancer in your family.

Susan Berry, of The Skin Cancer Foundation in New York City, says that you should see a doctor if you notice any changes in a mole, such as changes in color, size, thickness, texture or shape. Spots or growths that itch, hurt, crust, scab or seem to be eroding or dissolving also warrant attention. In the illustration shown here, the first mole is harmless; the others should be examined by a doctor.

Even if a mole looks suspicious, don't panic. Most moles are not cancerous. And even if a mole is malignant, if detected early, the growth can be removed quickly and painlessly by a doctor before it has a chance to affect surrounding skin.

people this measure is enough to prevent trouble. Others aren't so lucky, including those who react to balsam of Peru (a mild antiseptic) and certain forms of formaldehyde, among other ingredients. So manufacturers who wish to market a product as hypoallergenic must test it on many people with sensitive skin. For example, a spokesperson for one leading manufacturer of hypoallergenic cosmetics said that the company tests its products by repeatedly applying them, under a dermatologist's supervision, to the skin of 600 allergy-prone people. Only those products that trigger no reaction within the test period—usually several weeks—are marketed.

In order to develop hypoallergenic versions of skin care products and makeup, manufacturers rely on chemists and dermatologists to develop safe ingredients and test new formulas. Dermatologists say that, in general, the bigger the company, the more time and money is spent on research and the less apt their products are to cause trouble.

Even if you react to a hypoallergenic product, some manufacturers will take extra steps to help you solve the problem. Almay, for example, says it will provide your physician with a product guide that spells out all possible causes of an unusual reaction to any of its products. And Almay's director of professional services and director of medical affairs are available for advice. When feasible, the company will go so far as to custom-mix a formula free of the troublesome ingredients.

HOUSEWORK DERMATITIS

Detergents, shampoos and even some foods can also wreak havoc with your skin. To speed healing and prevent repeat outbreaks, Stephen M. Schleicher, M.D., of The Dermatology Center in Philadelphia, offers the following tips:

- Wash your hands with lukewarm (not hot) water and as little soap as possible (the milder, the better). Rinse thoroughly and dry gently.
- Clean the inside of your rings

A Natural Way to Prevent Scars

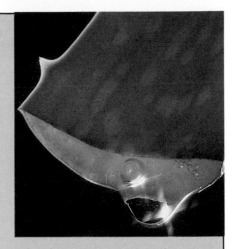

Say you fall off your bike and skin your knee. Or cut yourself on broken glass. Or burn your hand on a hot pan. Mishaps like these can leave your skin permanently scarred—but rubbing the wound with fresh aloe vera juice and vitamin E oil may prevent that from happening.

How? The juice from an aloe vera plant contains lectins, proteins that help blood cells clump together. Lectins also stimulate the production of lymphocytes, white blood cells that help fight infection.

When vitamin E is put on a wound, it speeds "granulation"—the formation of new, tiny veins that help patch skin together. With all these factors at work at once, a scar is less likely.

To apply aloe vera, slice off a section of the plant, which is easily grown at home. (Only fresh aloe vera gel works. Stabilizers and other ingredients in commercial preparations often deactivate aloe's special properties.) Squeeze out a teaspoon or so of its thick juice and mix with the oil from 2 or 3 vitamin E capsules (or ½ teaspoon of vitamin E oil from a bottle). Apply the mixture to a clean wound, 1 to 3 times a day, for a month. (If necessary, cover the injured area with a plastic adhesive bandage to prevent the mixture from staining your clothes.)

frequently with a brush. Soak them overnight in a solution of 1 tablespoon ammonia to 2 cups of water, then rinse thoroughly.
- Pour or measure solutions of detergent, solvents and stain removers carefully to avoid splashing onto unprotected skin.
- Don't peel or squeeze oranges, lemons or grapefruit with bare hands. Full-strength citric acid can irritate sensitive skin.

In short, the less direct contact between your skin and strong compounds of any kind, the better. Nia Terezakis, M.D., known for her "less

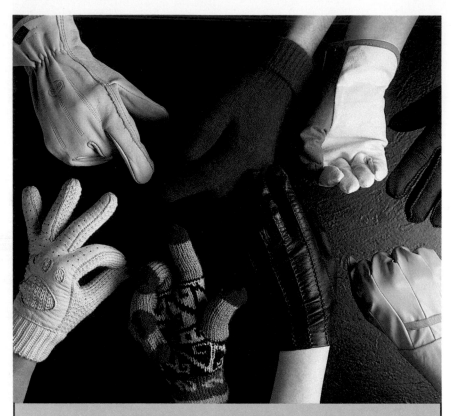

Put on the Gloves

Because your hands slosh around in hot water, detergents and solvents—and knuckle under to cold, dry winds—they're apt to chap or break out in a red, itchy rash long before other parts of your skin act up. And that's why gloves were invented.

Always wear gloves when venturing out into the cold, to keep your hands soft and beautiful even in harsh weather. When washing dishes and doing other household chores, wear cotton gloves (available at pharmacies) topped with plastic gloves (such as Playtex heavy-duty gloves). Unlined rubber gloves aren't quite as good—they tend to irritate sensitive skin and cause rashes. If your gloves get wet inside, pull them off immediately. Turn the gloves inside, out and rinse them under hot water. Let them dry, then sprinkle plastic gloves with cornstarch before wearing them again— damp gloves can irritate sensitive skin.

To protect your hands from stains and irritation, slip on gloves whenever you:
• Apply hair dye
• Polish shoes, windows or silverware
• Wax floors, cars or furniture
• Work with solvents and stain removers such as turpentine

is better" philosophy of skin care, offers these additional tips:

- For laundry, use low-suds detergents without additives. Fabric softeners, foaming agents and other cleaning boosters can rile sensitive skin.
- Wash any new fabrics a few times to remove chemical treatments. Wrinkle-resistant agents in wash-and-wear fabrics tend to irritate sensitive skin.
- Wear as much 100 percent cotton clothing as possible, and use cotton sheets and pillowcases.

If your skin breaks out despite these precautions, soothe it by soaking in a cool or tepid colloidal bath, made with colloidal oatmeal (available in drugstores), skim milk, powdered milk or baking soda. Hot baths make itching worse.

If you can't stand the itching, apply shake lotions such as calamine lotion or milk of bismuth.

ADULT ACNE: CAUSES AND CURES

Common knowledge holds that blemishes are caused by chocolate and greasy food, by dirt, by too much sex or not enough sex and by psychological hangups. None of these is true, says James E. Fulton, M.D., Ph.D., director of the Acne Research Institute in Newport Beach, California. Nor does oily skin cause acne. True, most people who have acne also have oily skin. But you can have very oily skin and never sprout a single pimple. Acne, he says, is caused by a genetic quirk that prompts your pores to behave differently from the pores of people who do not have acne. Acne is *not* your fault.

The process itself is complex, and even doctors who've studied acne for years don't completely understand it. But acne flareups are basically triggered by dihydrotestosterone (DHT), a souped-up form of testosterone, a hormone secreted by both men and women (although men secrete about ten times more than women do). DHT stimulates your sebaceous glands to produce oil. At

Skin-Saving Tips for Sports Enthusiasts

People who play hard at sports have skin care needs all their own. Vigorous movements, exposure to sun and weather and increased perspiration can set you up for blisters, rashes and other annoying skin ailments. Play hard, but play it safe: Follow these tips.

Skin Ailment	Sport Source	Symptoms	First Aid	Skin Savers
Athlete's foot	Sport shoes that lock in sweat. Exposure in the locker room.	Fungus causes peeling, itchy blisters between toes.	Soak in milk and ice water. Apply zinc ointment or antifungal agent like tolnaftate.	Keep feet dry; wear absorbent cotton socks. Dust with cornstarch. Wear thongs in locker room.
Bikini bottom	Prolonged sitting in damp swimsuit or in hot tubs.	Infected wet blisters on buttocks.	Rub area with alcohol. Let skin air-dry.	Change suit periodically. Get into dry clothes as soon as possible.
Black toenail ("tennis toe")	Short or narrow sport shoes. Sudden foot jamming in racquet sports.	Discoloration caused by bleeding under nail. Toenail may separate.	Soak in warm water; rest.	Fit shoes properly. Trim nails shorter. Wear cushiony socks.
Blisters	Friction between clothing or equipment and skin.	Fluid-filled skin sac. May become infected.	Clean, apply antiseptic, prick edge of blister with sterile needle. Do not remove skin flap; cover with bandage. Air-dry often.	Fit shoes and socks properly. Use absorbent powder to keep feet dry. Tape vulnerable areas.
Calluses	Pressure points or prolonged rubbing with clothing or equipment in tennis, rowing, sailing, gymnastics.	Thickening of skin on hands, feet. Protects skin against blisters.	Gently smooth with pumice and moisturizer.	Use padding to relieve pressure.
Cold sores ("fever blisters")	Exertion in sunlight.	Dormant virus erupts into tiny red blisters around mouth.	At first sign apply ice. Lysine and lactobacillus (the bacteria found in yogurt) have been found helpful.	Keep lips dry. Use PABA sunscreen, zinc oxide before exercising in the sun.
Hives	Change in body temperature, exertion, stress, sunlight.	Histamine released causes itchy, raised rash.	Treat with antihistamines, vitamin C.	Avoid sudden changes in body temperature. Premedicate with antihistamines.
Prickly heat	Any sweat-producing activity.	Clogged sweat ducts create rash under breasts, behind knees, at elbows and at creases in thighs.	Vitamin C at each meal has been shown effective for some. Apply cortisone cream.	Keep skin cool, dry. Wear loose clothing. Dust with cornstarch. Peel off sweaty clothes after a workout.
Saddle sores	Long-distance bike riding or horseback riding.	Irritation or open sores on buttocks.	Wash and apply alcohol. Apply vitamin E or fresh aloe vera. Cover with moleskin.	Use chamois or sheepskin seat cover. Keep pants dry. Apply cornstarch to absorb moisture.

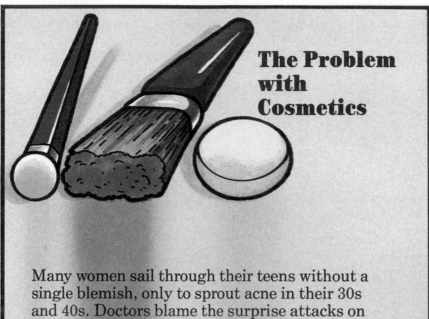

The Problem with Cosmetics

Many women sail through their teens without a single blemish, only to sprout acne in their 30s and 40s. Doctors blame the surprise attacks on certain lanolin compounds and other comedogenic (acne-promoting) ingredients in cosmetics. The ingredients in question don't necessarily *cause* acne, mind you—they simply aggravate acne-prone skin.

Because a cosmetic-induced blemish may take 6 months or more to surface, you may not connect the outbreak with daily, seemingly uneventful, use of cosmetics. You may even pile on *more* cosmetics to try to cover the problem.

To avoid or clear up cosmetic-induced acne, wear as little makeup as possible—and shop carefully for any makeup you do wear.

As a rule, water-based or glycerin-based cosmetics are least likely to instigate acne. The worst culprits are cosmetics that contain oils and certain other ingredients. Fortunately, cosmetic labels list ingredients in order of their proportion in the formula, so look for products that contain the least amount of these problem chemicals:

- Laureth-4 (a coconut oil derivative)
- Acetylated or ethoxylated lanolin (derivatives of sheepskin oil)
- Stearic acid and its derivatives (such as isopropyl myristate or butyl stearate)
- Sodium lauryl sulfate (an emulsifier)
- Octyl palmitate (a texturizer, often derived from palm oil)
- Decyl oleate (a lubricant and antifoam agent)
- Coal tar dyes D&C Red Nos. 4, 6, 19, 21, 27, 33 and 36 (found in nearly all blushers)

the same time, acne-prone skin produces hard, keratin-loaded skin cells at four to five times the normal rate. And certain kinds of bacteria, called anaerobes, thrive in pores, where there is no oxygen, and irritate surrounding tissue. Dead skin cells, bacteria and other debris commingle with oil to form thick plugs.

You can see why chocolate and sex have nothing to do with acne. Flareups may be triggered by any of a dozen factors, including menstrual cycles, birth control pills and stress. But aggravating factors only fuel an underlying condition.

Each blemish takes 90 days to form, beginning as a whitehead, or closed comedo. At that point, the bump may turn into a blackhead (open comedo), which may simply fall out on its own (with a little patience) or submit to pressure (with impatience). Blackheads are dark because as the plug forms, it picks up melanin as it forms and darkens further as the oily contents are exposed to oxygen on the surface. If the pore ruptures during the process, the plug may form a true pimple. If the pimple becomes inflamed, it can turn into a cyst the size of a large pea. Inflamed acne can leave scars long after the original blemishes have disappeared.

You may sport various stages of acne at any given time. Each one calls for a different type of attention, sort of like one-, two- or three-alarm fires.

COMING TO THE RESCUE

Five-alarm pimples always seem to erupt right before you're scheduled to take part in some event where you're highly visible, like having your passport picture taken. It's a rare person who can resist the temptation to squeeze a pimple, even knowing full well that digging and squeezing can lead to greater inflammation and possible scarring.

Dr. Fulton figures that as long as people are going to pick at their blemishes, they should learn to do it correctly. In fact, squeezing the right pimple at the right time in the right way can actually speed healing, stop tissue destruction and reduce scarring.

While cysts and immature, hard pimples are best left to a professional for treatment, Dr. Fulton says that blackheads are fair game. It's okay to go after a whitehead, too, provided it's reasonably close to the surface. You can even extract a mature pimple.

"A few days after you first notice a yellowish center developing in a pimple, pus has moved up to the surface, bringing the impaction with it," says Dr. Fulton. "Then it is ripe for extraction."

Here's Dr. Fulton's battle plan: Use benzoyl peroxide for three weeks or more. (This is a *must*.) Available at drugstores, benzoyl peroxide will open up the pores and loosen plugs. It is the cornerstone of Dr. Fulton's treatment program for mild to moderate acne. Similar in action to hydrogen peroxide, benzoyl peroxide releases oxygen into the pores, killing anaerobic bacteria. Dr. Fulton thinks benzoyl peroxide controls acne better than the antibiotic tetracycline (though he sometimes uses benzoyl peroxide and antibiotics together). Benzoyl peroxide lotions also peel the skin, loosening plugs.

Surprisingly, the potency of a benzoyl peroxide product is not necessarily related to the amount of the solution it contains but to the way it's combined with other ingredients. For example, a 5 percent benzoyl peroxide product in a water-based gel could be stronger than a 10 percent product in an oil base. Also, some benzoyl peroxide products contain acne-*promoting* oils such as isopropyl myristate. You could use them forever with no improvement. (See "The Problem with Cosmetics" for other ingredients to avoid.)

If applied lightly, benzoyl peroxide can be worn under makeup. The directions on acne medications usually instruct people who use benzoyl peroxide to apply it to "the affected area." Most people assume that means they should dab it right on the pimple and nowhere else. What you really need to do, says Dr. Fulton, is apply it to the pimples and to the areas in which you are *likely* to break out, be it the face, neck, back or shoulders. (Avoid applying benzoyl peroxide to the eye area and sensitive areas around the nose and mouth, which are easily irritated. And if you use it on the neck, use a milder solution.) The idea is to head off breakouts before they bloom.

Thirty minutes before you apply this peeling lotion, wash your face with soap and water. To build up your tolerance, begin with a mild solution such as Cuticura, or Noxzema BP or Porox 7, and work up to stronger lotions three or four days after peeling has slowed down. At first apply benzoyl peroxide for 2 to 3 hours each day, washing it off afterward. (People with very sensitive skin should only leave it on for 15 to 30 minutes.) Then work up to twice a day and overnight.

While benzoyl peroxide is effective, you should use this technique cautiously. For one thing, the strength of the solution and the length of the time you leave it on should depend on the type of skin you have and who you are. A young person may react differently than someone who's older; someone with oily skin may react differently than someone with dry skin. Also, some people may be allergic to it. (Your clothes can be "allergic" to it too—remember it's a *peroxide,* a bleach.) So make sure you consult your dermatologist before using this treatment. After two to four months the blemishes may begin to clear up, says Dr. Fulton.

There are effective ways to manually extract a pimple. But choose your weapon carefully. Of the various comedo extractors sold in drugstores, Dr. Fulton feels that the Schaumberg extractor is the best. If you must squeeze a blemish with your fingers, wash your hands thoroughly, as though you were scrubbing for surgery. Pierce the whitehead with a thin, sterilized needle. (You should skip this step with blackheads, of course.) Wrap the padded tips of your fingers with tissue and apply gentle pressure to either side. If you have long fingernails, trim them so you won't risk scarring your skin permanently.

If the blackhead or plug doesn't pop out easily on the first couple of tries, don't force it.

An Answer to Acne: A Low-Iodine Diet

Clearing up a long-standing case of acne may be as simple as avoiding foods high in iodine. Oil glands excrete excess iodine that can irritate pores, so a steady diet of foods containing even moderate amounts of the mineral can trigger one flareup after another if you're prone to breakouts.

There's no need to eliminate every last trace of iodine from your diet, however. In fact, it would be dangerous to your health. Just be sure that any multivitamin or mineral tablet you take is free of iodine, and steer clear of the high-iodine foods listed below.

Food	Iodine Content (parts per million)
Kelp	1,020
Beef liver	325
Asparagus	169
Turkey	132
Broccoli	90
Onions, white	82
Tortilla chips	80
Iodized salt	54
Potato chips, salted	40
Sea salt	30

The Ten Best Things You Can Do for Your Skin

one

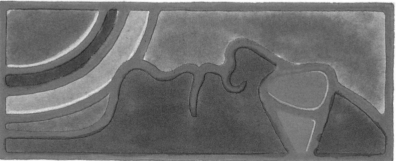

If you smoke, try to quit. If you don't smoke, give yourself a gold star. Studies have shown that people who smoke have deeper and sharper wrinkles at the outer corners of their eyes (crow's feet) and that the skin on the backs of their necks takes on a cobblestone appearance. Smokers' skin also tends to be pale and sallow rather than pink and rosy. And, apparently, smoking makes your skin more vulnerable to sun-induced damage. So if you quit smoking today, you can stop wrinkles in their tracks.

two

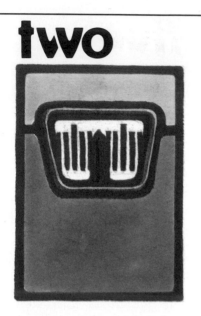

Pick a weight that suits you best and stick to it. Crash dieting or yo-yo fluctuations in weight—losing and gaining 20 or 30 pounds again and again—stretch your tissues, leaving your skin saggy and wrinkled.

three

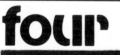

Use moisturizers and foundation makeups that contain sunscreen. "Unquestionably, women in their 40s, 50s and 60s who've used sunscreens look years younger than those who don't," says one dermatologist.

four

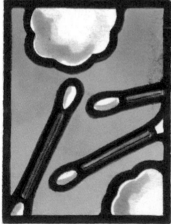

Use cotton swabs and cleanser to wipe away smudges around your eyes. Tissues and paper towels are too coarse and will stretch fragile skin, exaggerating lines or crepeyness.

five

Turn down the heat and turn on the humidifier. A cool, moist environment—50 to 60 percent humidity—is most comfortable for your skin. In winter, skin exposed to superheated indoor air and chilling winds can lose water up to 140 times as fast as it does in humid weather, leaving it dry and parched.

six

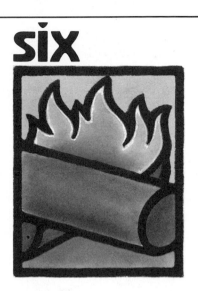

Keep a comfortable distance from heat sources like open fireplaces and wood stoves, and never use a sun reflector to speed up your tan. Heat amplifies damage from the environment.

seven

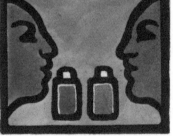

Choose skin care products according to your skin type. For example, using an oil-based makeup instead of a water-based product on oily skin can promote blackheads. Using an alcohol-based astringent on dry skin can dry your face even more.

eight

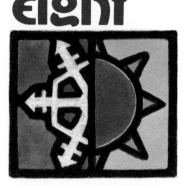

Change your moisturizer with the seasons. In winter, when your skin is apt to be exposed to dry air, you need a creamier moisturizer. In warm weather, use a lighter-textured lotion that vanishes into the skin and allows it to breathe.

ten

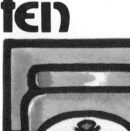
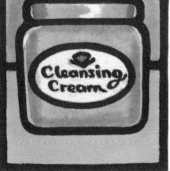

Never go to sleep at night without removing every trace of makeup—except maybe on New Year's Eve. Habitually sleeping with a layer of dirt, debris and dead skin cells stuck to your face will leave your complexion looking muddy and dull.

nine

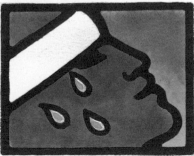

If you exercise hard enough to work up a sweat, remove your foundation or makeup so perspiration doesn't have to fight its way out of your pores.

3

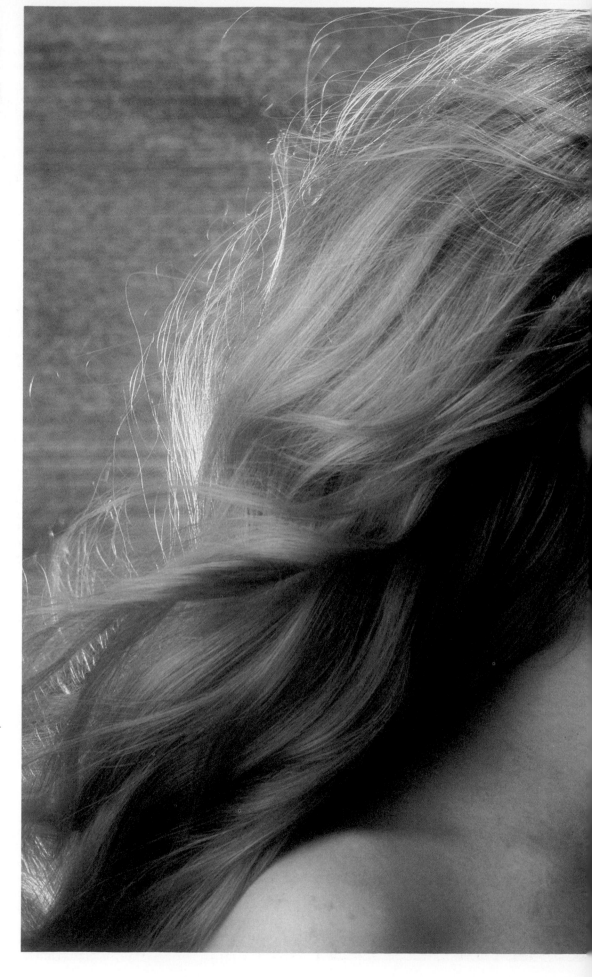

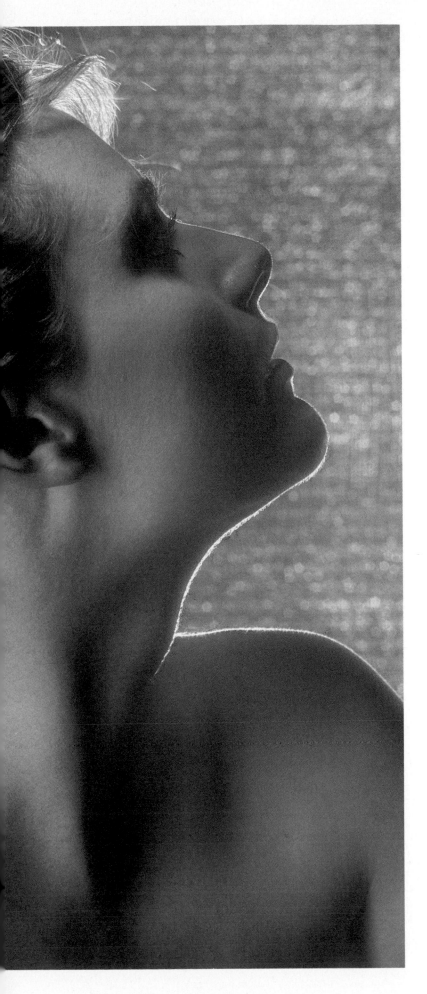

The Secrets of Healthy Hair

How to pamper your hair so it will look better than ever. Shiny. Luxuriant. Touchable.

Can you predict how your hair will behave each day as soon as you hear the weather report? Flyaway when the air is cold and dry? Frizzy when it's humid? If so, you can imagine the *cumulative* effects that sun, wind and water can have on the way your hair looks and feels. (Of course, other factors—styling, diet, stress—can also "weather" your hair.) Cultivating beautiful, healthy hair is a matter of combating the collective effects of every form of weather-beating your hair takes. To show you how to do that is the purpose of this chapter. And the first step is to understand your hair's behavior, starting at the cellular level.

If you were to view a cross-section of a single hair under a microscope you wouldn't see a solid, uniform shaft but three distinct layers. At the center, forming the innermost core, you'd see a column of soft, loosely packed cells, called the medulla. A thicker layer of tightly packed, elongated cells, the cortex, surrounds the medulla and gives hair its strength and color. The cuticle, a layer of tough cells that overlap each other like roof shingles, coats the hair shaft.

Each hair grows out of a pore in the skin called a follicle. At any given time, about 85 percent of your hair is growing. The remaining hairs are either resting between growth spurts or are about to be shed. Each hair has a life cycle of anywhere from three to ten years and grows at an average rate of ½ inch per month. Simple calculation shows, for example, that hair 12 inches long is two years old. That's two years of weathering, of tugging and twisting by combs, brushes and other grooming tools—all of which can roughen the hair shaft and affect how your hair looks and behaves.

For example, nothing brings out your hair's brilliant highlights the way warm, glistening sunshine does. Yet people who've studied hair under microscopes report that when the hair shaft absorbs the ultraviolet beams of sunlight—the invisible light waves—certain chemical changes that occur break down hair protein, or keratin. Over time, that weakens hair. Also, light hair yellows and dark hair fades—much like a wool rug that lies near a sunny window.

Wind, too, can take its toll. Sun and wind together can strip off the protective outer cuticle. On healthy hair, cuticle cells lie flat. Anything that roughens the cuticle will lift those cells and leave hair dull, damaged and unmanageable. Even air pollution can "weather" hair!

Swimming—in fresh water, salt water or chlorinated pools—can also hurt your hair. Water acts as a catalyst, speeding up the damaging effects of sun and wind. But it can also do a job by itself. Salt water dries hair; so does chlorine. So when your hair is wet, you want to dry it quickly, right? Well, blow dryers can actually singe your hair. And there are plenty of other man-made assaults that rival anything Mother Nature has to offer.

Permanent wave treatments, bleaches and hair dyes contain strong chemicals that can strip away natural oils and roughen the hair surface if they're not used very carefully. In fact, almost *anything* that comes in contact with your hair has the power to damage it, robbing it of its natural luster and bounce. The list includes not only harmful elements but also beauty products that can be misused, such as brushes, combs, shampoos, conditioners, scissors, rollers, curling irons, hair spray, mousses, gels, straighteners and relaxers. Whew!

How long does it take for hair to feel (and look) "under the weather"? A few months. In one laboratory study, reported in *Cosmetics and Toiletries,* researchers examined both bleached and waved hair (some brown, some blond) under natural conditions—12 weeks of exposure to the sun during July, August and September. The hair became progressively weaker as the summer wore on. And blond hair suffered more than brown.

Apparently, melanin (the pigment responsible for a tan and the coloring of dark-skinned people) also protects brown hair from the sun. Researchers also found that weather affected bleached or waved hair more severely than untreated hair, regardless of its basic color. That's because chemical treatments add to the damage caused by sun, wind, salt and other environmental onslaughts.

Hair is a barometer of the weather in your inner environment, too. Philip Kingsley, a trichologist (hair care specialist) in New York, explains that changes occurring during the menstrual cycle, pregnancy, menopause, aging and stress all affect the color, texture and manageability of hair. A woman's hair may be the least manageable just before or after her period. If her hair is usually a little greasy, it may be exceptionally greasy at that time. If she has dandruff, her scalp may flake more than usual. Hair also tends to grow finer and dry out with age in both men and women, whether or not it turns gray.

All those effects are more obvious at the tips of the hair shaft than near the scalp, since the ends have been around longer and have been exposed to more weather.

With all these enemies, the more you do to pamper and protect your hair, the better. The most important steps are often quite simple—like shielding your hair from sun and wind by wearing a hat in winter *and* summer. Or using a conditioner to protect against drying. Or choosing a perm that curls your hair gently. Or drying your hair at settings closer to the temperature of a warm breeze than of a blowtorch.

Your hair deserves the same respect and care you'd give any delicate, fine possession. Start with gentle brushing.

EASY-DOES-IT COMBING AND BRUSHING

A comb and brush do more than divide and conquer strands of hair. Brushing helps to clean your hair by loosening and removing dust, dirt and dead cells and helps to distribute oil along the hair shaft.

Take it easy, though. Hard brushing—or using the wrong brush

(continued on page 36)

What the Weather Can Do to Your Hair

Each hair shaft consists of a soft, inner core (the medulla), wrapped in a thicker cell layer (the cortex) that's covered by a layer of protective outer cells, called the cuticle. Weather and improper hair care can roughen and strip off the outer layer, weakening your hair and changing the way it looks and feels.

Under an electron microscope, new hair looks healthy and undamaged at the root. The cuticle is smooth, the hair shaft strong.

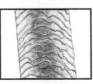

Sun, wind, water and air pollution dry the hair and roughen the surface.

Teasing, blow-drying and perms or colorings damage and further weaken hair.

Hair splits and frays at the tip, where the hair has been exposed to the most "bad weather."

The Right Comb and Brush for You

Some combs and brushes are better for your hair than others. Combs made of vulcanite (hard rubber) are usually kinder to your hair than most plastic or metal combs. Brush bristles should be long, smooth and blunt or rounded at the tip. (Replace your brush if it has split bristles, which can damage hair.) Here are a few examples of top-notch brushes and combs.

Mock tortoise-shell comb, with a wide-toothed end for detangling and a fine-toothed end for styling.

Air-flow vent brush. Open spaces allow air from a blow dryer to flow freely during styling.

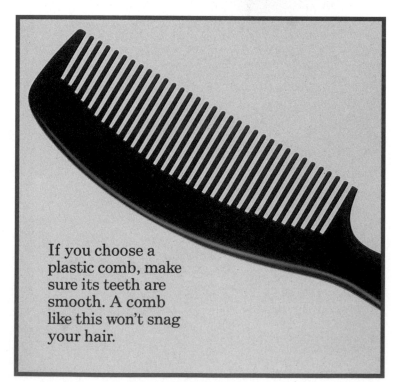

If you choose a plastic comb, make sure its teeth are smooth. A comb like this won't snag your hair.

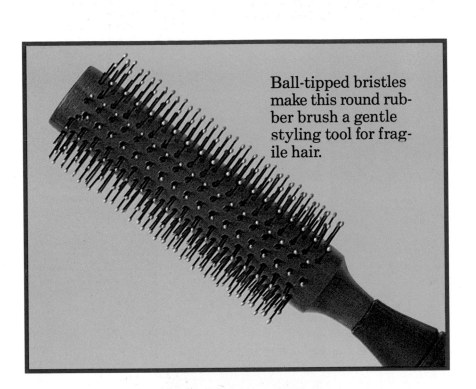

Ball-tipped bristles make this round rubber brush a gentle styling tool for fragile hair.

Shampoo Your Brush and Comb

To keep your comb and brush as clean as your hair, wash them once a month (more often, if you have oily hair). Here's how:

- Remove loose hair strands from your brush with a wide-toothed comb.
- Immerse the comb and brush (bristles only, if the brush is wood) in warm, soapy water. Shampoo works well. For added cleaning power, add a few drops of ammonia to the cleaning solution.
- Rinse in clear, warm water and shake out gently.
- Dry your comb and brush handle with a towel, then air-dry both on a towel, with brush bristles facing down.

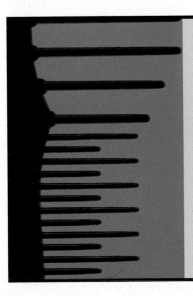

Saw-cut comb of black vulcanized rubber. A static-free detangler for all hair types.

Flexible styling brush. Angled bristles are embedded in a resilient rubber base.

or comb—can strip away the outer, protective cells of hair, leaving the soft inner cortex vulnerable to further damage by the weather and chemical treatments. Too-vigorous brushing can also uproot hairs that are in the resting stage of growth and therefore are not firmly anchored in the follicle. Hard brushing also can irritate the scalp.

As you might expect, teasing or backcombing can be brutal: Combing against the grain ruffles the hair's outer cuticle. While this may give the hair added body, it leaves it dull and ragged in the process. Teasing also creates tangles, which lead to further tugging, pulling and breakage. If your hair is dry and brittle to begin with, or breaks easily, teasing is the coup de grace.

If you customarily tease your hair, consider a root perm or other means of adding lift and volume to your hair instead.

Never brush your hair when it's wet. Period. Hair stretches more easily when wet, and it can stretch only so far before it snaps and breaks. So wet hair is weak hair. A wide-toothed rubber comb is the best tool for parting your hair and working out tangles after a shampoo. If your hair is long or curly (and therefore prone to tangles), begin by combing through the 2 or 3 inches closest to the ends first, then gradually work your way closer to the scalp, section by section. Don't try to rush the job by starting at the scalp and combing straight through from top to bottom, unless you have short hair. That only tends to make big knots out of small ones.

Believe it or not, there's a lot of controversy over what type of combs and brushes are best. Some hairdressers swear by natural boar-bristle brushes; dermatologists and certain scientific experts claim that boar-bristle brushes are useless or even harmful. Some people use nothing but wooden-handled brushes or tortoise-shell combs and wouldn't touch plastic with a 10-foot pole (wooden, of course). The fact is, the kind of comb or brush you use isn't half as important as *how* you brush.

"No matter what type of brush you buy, you'll have problems if you brush wrong," says William J. Ware, former president of the National Hairdressers and Cosmetologists Association. "Brush your hair in sections, starting at the nape of the neck and working your way to the crown, brushing the portion nearest the end first.

"That technique is especially helpful to people with oily hair," Ware says. "Even if you brush your hair four or five times a day, that technique minimizes oiliness if you're using a natural-bristle brush."

For most people, brushing two or three times a day should be adequate—just enough to tidy up. *Do* brush your hair before each shampoo to whisk away surface dirt and free hair of tangles.

SHAMPOO FINESSE

Shampoo carries more mystique than any other hair care product. According to the ads, getting hair squeaky clean is no longer enough to ask of a product. We've been told that shampoo can make limp, oily hair light and fluffy, with lots of volume; balance the acid-base levels; cure dandruff and other scalp problems—and even improve our love lives!

That's a tall order for a couple teaspoons of limpid gel. Just how much can we realistically expect a shampoo to do? And what makes one shampoo different from another?

Shampoo is a special breed of detergent, designed to clean hair and hair alone. Don't let the term *detergent* scare you: Detergents are generally *milder* than soap and kinder to your hair. Combined with various foaming agents and other ingredients to help lift dirt off hair, shampoo can clean your hair more effectively than soap and water.

Cleaning is both a chemical and a mechanical process, so you need to use the right formula in the right way. In addition to the detergent, shampoos usually contain fragrances and other compounds that make the shampoo feel and smell appealing but have nothing to do with performance. It's more important to choose a shampoo designed for the type of hair you have—oily or dry, healthy or damaged, treated or untreated—than one that contains herbs, vitamins or other trendy ingredients.

Manufacturers formulate shampoos for different hair types and usually label them for "dry," "oily" or "normal" hair. The trick is to lift off excess oil without stripping hair of essential moisture and drying the scalp. Manufacturers strike this balance by regulating the strength or amount of detergent.

What kind of hair do you have?

Dry hair tends to split, break or frizz. Damaged hair is usually dry, especially at the ends. If your hair has been permed, colored or straightened, it's probably dry. Most people with hair that's coarsely textured have dry hair, although anyone is susceptible.

Oily hair tends to stick together; consequently, it looks limp and mats down. Oily hair doesn't hold a set well. It's often found in combination with dandruff. Oily hair gets oilier still in hot weather, increasing the need to shampoo.

Normal hair has a slight sheen, is only slightly oily, holds a set and bounces when clean. Ironically, most people have either oily or slightly dry hair, so "normal" hair isn't so normal after all.

Many shampoos claim to be "acid (or pH) balanced." That means

Shampoo Tips

- Brush your hair to loosen dirt.
- Wet your hair with warm water, loosening and separating it with your fingers so water can penetrate well.
- Mix shampoo with an equal amount of water.
- Work shampoo through your hair, separating the hair with your fingers as you lather *gently*. Rinse. Lather again—but only if your hair is very oily. (Otherwise, you could strip your hair of its natural oils.)
- Rinse thoroughly—for at least a full minute.

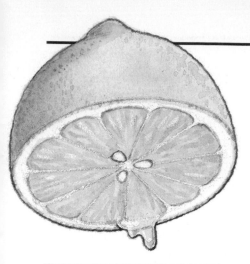

Water That's Hard on Your Hair

Calcium and magnesium in hard water react with shampoos that have soap in them to form an insoluble film—sort of like a "bathtub ring" on your hair.

To prevent this film's formation, add white vinegar or lemon juice to your rinse water. The acids will break down soapy film.

For an occasional treat, use distilled (mineral-free) water instead of tap water when you shampoo.

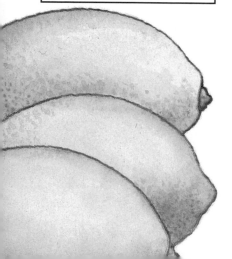

they're slightly acidic, just like human hair, which has a pH level of somewhere between 4.5 and 5.5. Alkaline shampoos are not as compatible with hair chemistry, so they can weaken hair shafts and increase the risk of damage from perms and other chemical treatments. (Most soap is alkaline, which is one of the reasons it makes a poor shampoo.)

Shampoos that are pH balanced, on the other hand, make hair shafts stronger and shinier and help to make hair easier to manage. So if your hair is the least bit damaged, choose a pH-balanced shampoo.

ARE SALON SHAMPOOS BETTER?

Many people are convinced that salon shampoos leave their hair cleaner and fluffier than home shampoos (see "Shampoo Tips" on page 37). There are several possible reasons for this. Salon attendants can use more "elbow grease," massaging shampoo in more thoroughly out of sheer mechanical advantage: They're working above your head. Salon shampoo brands are also more concentrated (that's why they cost more than supermarket or drugstore brands, which contain more water). And salon attendants rinse thoroughly.

"If shampoo leaves a film on your hair, it means either you're using too much or you're not rinsing thoroughly enough," Ware explains. "Many people think they need mounds of lather to get their hair clean. That's just for glamour. In fact, one salon brand produces no lather at all and does a fine job."

As for how often you should shampoo—once a week? daily? every other day?—ask three different hairdressers and you'll get three different answers.

The truth is, you should shampoo as often as *you* think you need to. It's a matter of personal aesthetics. In the South Sea islands, for example, oily hair is considered sexy. The oilier the hair, the more fertile a woman is thought to be. And, as it happens, oily hair is very remotely related to sex hormones, so there is a theoretical basis for that associa-

tion. But here in the United States, most people like their hair the way they like their souffles—light and fluffy, with lots of volume. So a lot of people shampoo daily. If you sweat heavily or pick up city soot or country dirt in your hair, you may sometimes have to shampoo twice in one day, no matter what type of shampoo you buy.

Don't be surprised if your favorite shampoo seems to leave your hair less bouncy after several months of satisfactory performance. No one is exactly sure why that seems to happen, but Rebecca Caserio, M.D., director of the hair clinic at the University of Pittsburgh School of Medicine, says that "shampoo fatigue" may be due to a buildup of proteins or other types of conditioning ingredients. Many people switch brands at that point, only to perceive an eventual drop in performance with the alternative shampoo a few months later. As buildup of one ingredient subsides, buildup of another can occur, according to Dr. Caserio.

DANDRUFF CONTROL MADE EASY

Everyone's scalp flakes somewhat—that's the scalp's way of shedding dead cells. If you shampoo regularly, the flakes are hardly noticeable. But when the stuff starts to look like snow flurries, you have dandruff. Your scalp may also be dry or oily and itch.

False dandruff is easy to control. Simply clear away the dead cells by shampooing more frequently than usual with your regular shampoo. True dandruff is a more severe condition. It consists of a *very* scaly scalp, often itchy and dry but sometimes oily. (Coupled with a rash, severe dandruff is known as seborrhea.) If you do have true dandruff, you can help control the problem by rinsing with an antiseptic solution, described in "Trouble-Free Hair—Easy Solutions to Tough Problems" on pages 54–55. If that doesn't work, you can try any one of a number of shampoos especially designed to control dandruff. They contain either sulfur, tar, salicylic acid, selenium or zinc pyrithione—or a combination of those compounds. You may have to try two or three brands to find one that works for you. (In case you haven't guessed by now, dandruff control is largely a matter of trial and error.)

Whatever you buy, read the directions: To be effective, many dandruff shampoos must be left on the scalp for several minutes.

Even when used correctly, all dandruff shampoos lose their effectiveness after about three months, no matter what the active ingredient. Skin cells develop a temporary resistance to the compound in question. Switching to a brand with a different active ingredient usually solves the problem.

THE SECRET OF SHINY HAIR

In order to shimmer with life, hair must be clean. But there's much more to shiny hair than using the right shampoo. Any soapy film left on the hair will leave it looking dull. A final rinse with a slightly acidic solution—such as 2 tablespoons of white vinegar, lemon juice or camomile tea diluted in a quart of water—will remove every trace of shampoo and leave hair shiny.

Smooth hair reflects light and looks shiny, while rough hair absorbs light and looks dull. So hair that's been roughed up by teasing, careless brushing, sun damage or chemical treatments can look dull.

Conditioners can restore some of that lost sheen. Applied after a shampoo, conditioners are substances—usually protein—that smooth over rough edges and fill in nicks and chips in the hair shafts. They restore luster to lifeless hair. Conditioners can also counteract dryness by sealing in moisture, which is what gives hair its elasticity and strength. Because they cling to the hair shaft, conditioners usually add body and protect the hair shaft from further damage. Conditioners also reduce static electricity, so they prevent tangles and leave hair more manageable.

After-shampoo conditioners are a boon to people who often swim in salt water or chlorinated pools, which can dry hair. They're also good for anyone who uses hot rollers, curling irons or blow dryers. Hair that's been permed, straightened or colored will hold up better with a little help from a conditioner. In short, practically everyone will notice that their hair is shinier and healthier looking if they regularly use an instant, after-shampoo conditioner.

With countless conditioners on the market, though, it may be hard to decide which ones are the best.

"Even I get confused, and I've been in the hair care business for 25 years," says Philip Kingsley. "But as a general rule, I'd say the thicker the conditioner, the better it will work.

"Also, look for 'quaternary' compounds, sometimes listed as quaternary 12 or 16 on the label," says Kingsley. Quaternary compounds are proteins that cling to the hair shaft, polishing the cuticle and softening the hair. "The higher the number, the greater the conditioning power," he adds.

One of the most unusual conditioners to come along in years contains reconstituted human hair. Don't let this ingredient put you off. Incorporated into hair care products, this "hydrolized human hair keratin protein" does wonders to restore sheen, give protection and aid in repairing damage. These products probably come as close to repairing damage as anything else hair technologists have developed so far. (You can read more about conditioning proteins in the section that discusses deep conditioners, later in this chapter.)

HOW TO CHOOSE A CONDITIONER THAT'S BEST FOR YOU

As with shampoos, you should choose a conditioner formulated for your hair type (dry, oily or normal), usually specified on the label. Otherwise, you risk overconditioning your hair, leaving it limp and lifeless.

"Conditioners for oily hair shouldn't contain any oil whatsoever," says Kingsley, "whereas conditioners for very dry hair need a certain amount of oil."

Some shampoos claim to condition as they clean. As you might expect, it's hard to clean away dirt and oil while adding oils and proteins at the same time. When one product tries to do two things at

A Sure Cure for Split Ends

A split end is a strand of hair that's frayed like a strand of yarn, exposing your hair's fragile inner layers.

To banish split ends, trim off the worst damage. Use an instant conditioner after *every* shampoo to prevent further damage and breakage. Deep-condition regularly, once a month or so.

Don't overdry your hair. And wear a hat outdoors to protect your hair from wind and sun.

What's Watt with Blow Dryers

Hand-held blow dryers pack a lot of power—over 1,200 watts for many models. That's enough energy to heat an iron or a toaster—and to cook your hair. To avoid *over*-drying your hair, look for a dryer with 1,200 watts of power or less. It will take a few minutes longer to dry your hair, but your gentleness will pay off in healthy luster.

Other features to look for in a blow dryer are:

- Switches to control temperature and speed.
- A diffuser attachment (the wider the better).
- Quiet operation (for comfort, because blow dryers are used so near the ears).
- An adapter switch for both 110-120-volt and 240-volt current for travel outside the U.S.

once, it tends to do each less effectively. A shampoo/conditioner is not as effective as a shampoo or a conditioner alone. You'll get much better results if you choose a shampoo on its own merits and follow up with an equally good conditioner.

To apply conditioner, squeeze excess water out of your hair. Pour about a tablespoon of conditioner into your palm (less if it's a salon-purchased, concentrated conditioner) and use your fingers to work it evenly through your hair. Allow the conditioner to work its magic for up to 60 seconds (read the directions for the exact time), then take at least 60 seconds to rinse *thoroughly* with warm water.

Creme rinses also give hair shine and reduce tangles because they coat the hair. Although they're not absorbed, creme rinses can help to protect the hair somewhat. For example, using either a creme rinse or a conditioner helps to protect your hair against the hot, desert-dry air of hair dryers. While some conditioners are marketed specifically for use with blow dryers, any conditioner will give you similar protection.

DEEP-CONDITION FOR LASTING BEAUTY

To rehabilitate hair that's been harmed by exposure to weather and chemical treatments—or to protect it beforehand—you have to deep-condition. That is, in addition to using an instant conditioner, you need to use a product that is designed to penetrate the hair shaft. (Instant and deep conditioners often share similar ingredients, formulated differently to perform differently.) Deep conditioners are left on the hair for 5 to 20 minutes, depending on the product you choose.

Because hair is basically protein and water, it would seem that protein could make the best deep conditioner. And, in fact, just such products have been developed.

"Protein is what gives hair bounce and hold," explains Dorothy Williams, vice president of education and research for Joi-Co Laboratories, in Gardena, California, a manufacturer of such a product. "Until

recently, manufacturers relied primarily on collagen (from animal skin) and keratin (from hooves and horns), labeled 'hydrolized animal protein.' But Joi-Co and others now offer conditioners containing hydrolized human hair keratin protein.

"Human hair keratin protein has a low molecular weight and therefore can penetrate the hair shaft rather than lie on the surface," says Ms. Williams. "In that way, they go one step further than other proteins to actually reconstruct the hair. And you don't need much—the hair absorbs only what it needs."

For many years, hot oil treatments have been promoted as a deep-conditioning technique. A *little* oil is good—it helps to seal in hair's natural moisture. But trying to condition by saturating the hair with oil is nonsense.

"Hot oil treatments *soften* the hair," says Ms. Williams, "but they don't help to retain moisture or protect against damage from weather and chemical pollution. And they certainly don't reconstruct the hair. To really reconstruct the hair, you need protein, perhaps with a little bit of oil if your hair is dry."

The best deep conditioners are those recommended by informed hairdressers. Certain ingredients, including botanicals, waxes or plasticizers, when not properly formulated to be shampoo-soluble, can leave hair shiny at first but with repeated use can leave it the consistency of chewing gum. Unfortunately, you can't tell which conditioners contain these potential troublemakers simply by reading the labels. The damage won't show up until you use the product for several weeks, and by then it's too late. To avoid disaster, trust a knowledgeable hairdresser's advice.

How often you deep-condition depends on how much sun, wind, water, heat and other elements you subject your hair to.

"I recommend a deep-conditioning treatment once a week, at least," says Kingsley. "And I'd certainly suggest a conditioning session *before* you head for the beach."

Conditioning is a must for people who perm or color their hair. Ditto for those who use straighteners.

(continued on page 44)

How to Trim Your Own Bangs

When your bangs fall into your eyes before the rest of your hair needs a trim, you can cut them yourself, with good-looking results.

Start with damp (not wet) hair. Use sharp scissors. Comb your hair straight back off your forehead. Then, using your comb and fingers, bring down a fine layer of hair. Taking just a few hairs at a time, hold the scissors vertically and trim the bangs. Continue to bring down additional fine layers, trimming as you go.

This technique may sound strange, but cutting hair at this angle will shorten your bangs and thin them at the same time. This technique is better than a blunt, horizontal cut because vertical snips give you a slightly uneven, "grown-in" look. Mistakes are less obvious and easier to remedy than with a straight horizontal cut, too. To slim a round face, leave your bangs longer at the sides. To add width to a slim, long face, cut your bangs farther back at the temples.

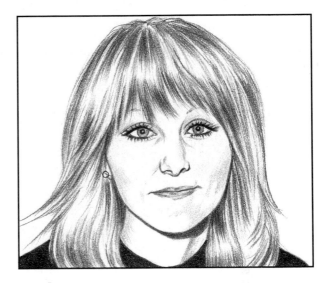

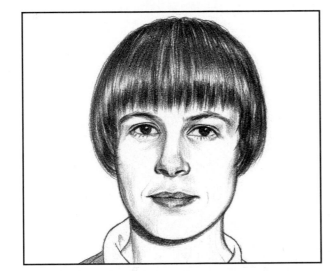

How to Choose the 'Do for You

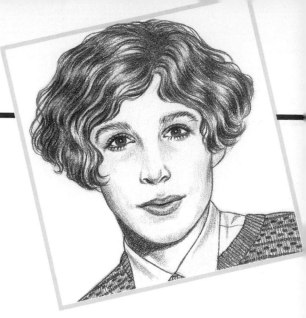

In any given year, a number of vastly different hairdos will be in style. You can choose to wear your hair long, short, curly, straight, pinned up or pulled back. Of course, few people have the perfectly oval face and balanced features that look good in *any* hairstyle. The style you choose should make the most of your very best features and play down your not-so-great features. Here are some guidelines.

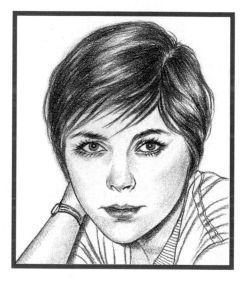

Too Round, "Baby Face"

A side part draws the viewer's eye diagonally, slimming and lengthening a face that's too round or full.

Thin Face

Curls or fullness at sides create horizontal lines, widening a long, thin face.

Large Nose

A full hairstyle or upswept crown deemphasizes the profile; the nose becomes less noticeable.

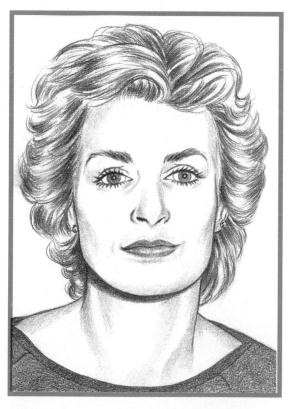

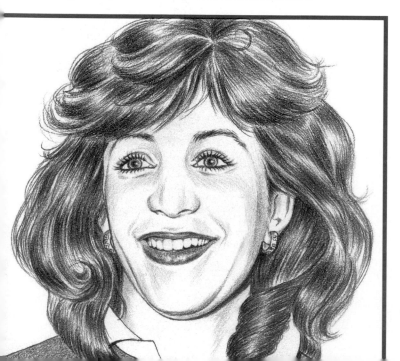

Sharp, Angular Features

A wavy or curly hairstyle will soften "chiseled" cheekbones, nose or other angular features.

42

High Forehead

The horizontal line of full bangs can obscure the forehead and balance the face.

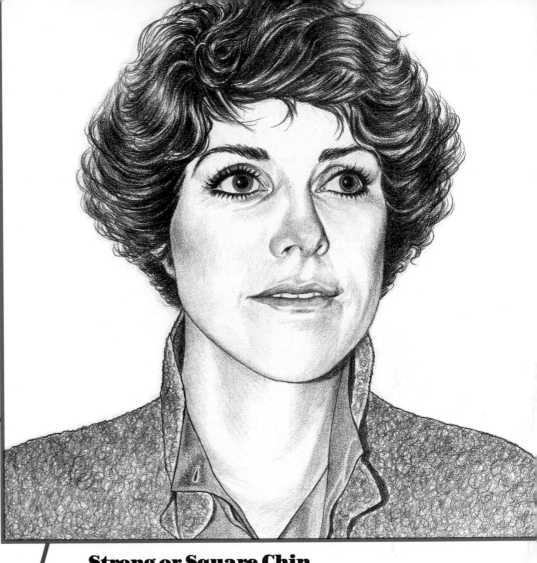

Strong or Square Chin

Short hair, with soft curls or fullness at the crown, draws the line of sight upward, away from the chin.

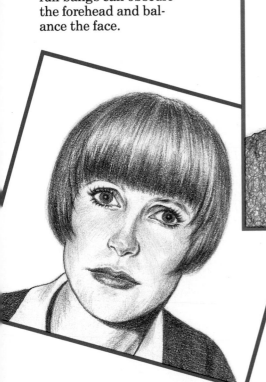

Narrow Chin

Long hair, with fullness at the chinline, balances a receding chin or narrow jawline.

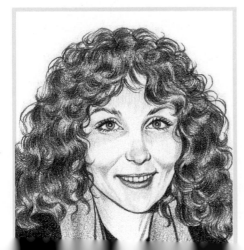

Low Forehead

Vertical lines and soft fullness at crown open up and lengthen the face.

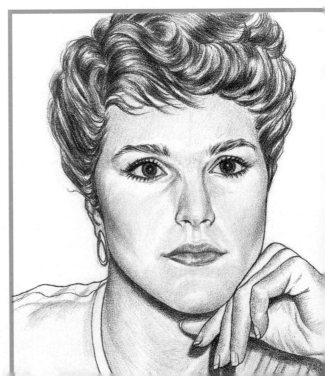

Hot Rollers: Better Than Ever

If you own hot rollers (electrically heated curlers that wave your hair in minutes) that are more than 2 or 3 years old, you might want to invest in a newer model. Today's hot rollers are more versatile—and kinder to your hair—than ever.

Some models are designed to accommodate all roller sizes so you can easily change your look from straight to curly or anything in between.

Some also offer universal voltage (120 to 240) for use outside the United States.

The most important feature to look for, though, is a velvet surface. The velvet acts as a buffer between your hair and the rod's heated inner core. That's a blessing to hair that's dry or slightly damaged from perms or bleaches and thus particularly vulnerable to heat. Fine or delicate hair rolls up more easily on velvet-wrapped rods, avoiding the pulls and tangles that metal or plastic spiked rods inflict.

"People don't realize that hair that's undergone more than one chemical treatment can get so dried out that it feels spongy when wet," says hair expert William Ware.

Use a conditioner formulated for chemically treated hair. And be sure to thoroughly rinse out any deep conditioners before you shampoo. Otherwise, the residue will leave hair dull and limp.

DRY, DON'T FRY, YOUR HAIR

Hair is weakest when it's wet. If you rub it vigorously with a towel, the strands are apt to break. Instead, blot your hair gently with a soft towel or terrycloth mittens. (Mittens work especially well on very long hair.)

Depending on your hairstyle, you may then simply fluff out your hair with your fingers and let it air-dry naturally. In fact, some curly or short hairstyles look *better* if air-dried. (Incidentally, you won't get a cold or pneumonia from going out in the cold with wet hair. That's a myth.)

Blow dryers can add lift and volume to hair. But use them *carefully*! Frequent steady blasts of their superheated air can parch your hair, leaving it brittle and lifeless. Some quick math says that 12-inch-long hair will have endured approximately 60 hours of intense heat if blown dry daily over its two-year life span. That's more than enough heat to leave hair dry and dull and the scalp flaky.

If you must blow-dry, take some precautions.

- Don't blow-dry hair that's sopping wet. Air-dry or blot first.
- Never hold a dryer closer than 6 inches from your hair.
- Keep the dryer moving constantly, to avoid singeing hair in spots.
- When your hair is half dry, bend over and continue to dry with your hair hanging toward the floor. That gives added lift to hair *and* prevents overdrying the outer strands.
- Stop when your hair is still slightly damp.

Because you can control those factors more easily with hand-held dryers, they're kinder to hair than hood or bonnet dryers.

SCISSORS-HAPPY

Unless you're a modern-day Rapunzel, you'll have your hair cut from time to time, be it for a whole new look or for regular maintenance trims. Some hairstyles begin and end with the cut. But even if you perm or set your hair, how it's cut will determine how good it will look.

Long hair has unmistakable appeal—it feels glamorous and sexy. But few people truly look their best in long hair—say, shoulder length or longer. If your hair is thin or limp, it will tend to look straggly. Even if it's thick or coarse, lots of volume can result in a shapeless mass unless it is cut correctly.

Consider, too, that long hair is old hair, and unless it's *very* healthy—no dryness or breakage—chances are you'll look better in short hair. In other words, it's easier to look good with short, healthy hair than with long, unruly or dull hair. Cut correctly, hair that's chin length or shorter can accentuate bone structure (and even reveal some you may never have noticed). Shorter still, hair can draw attention to your eyes and "elongate" your neck. (The exceptions: very large, big-boned women; women with wide necks, double chins, receding chins or big jaws. Longer hair will camouflage those features to some degree.)

Gray hair also looks better short. All hair tends to thin with age, and gray hair changes texture—sometimes becoming coarser. As a result, hair just doesn't behave the way it did earlier in life. A short haircut can keep gray hair looking fresh and perky.

Admittedly, going from long hair to short takes courage, but it has several advantages. If you're the least bit athletic, short hair is less of a nuisance and is easier to keep tidy. If you often travel, you won't have to lug a lot of hair care equipment with you. And wearing your hair short can save precious time if you lead a busy life.

HOW TO FIND A HAIR SALON THAT WON'T DISAPPOINT YOU

Once you've decided to change your hairstyle, the twinges of apprehension begin. They may be compounded if you're changing hairstylists, too. Salon visits don't have to be a game of chance, though. A little advance preparation can calm "salon jitters," whether you're simply getting a trim or undergoing a complete makeover.

Use Pictures to Lessen the Confusion. Make a habit of skimming magazines for pictures of hairstyles that appeal to you, even if you're not planning a salon visit in the near future. That way, you won't have to make a decision under pressure. But more important, a picture will spell out exactly what you have in mind, with little room for misunderstanding. If you want your hair short, for example, a picture will show the stylist whether you mean chin length, above your ears or somewhere in between. Likewise, if you want curls, a picture tells the stylist whether you want big, relaxed curls or tight little ringlets.

Bring pictures of more than one style, if you can, in case a particular style you admire isn't right for your bone structure or hair type.

It may also be helpful to browse through your family photo albums to refresh your memory about hair styles you liked—or hated—in the past.

Interview the Stylist. If you've never been to the salon, make a preliminary appointment to discuss your plans. A consultation of this sort can build your confidence on your first visit to a salon. Discuss your hair type, the style you want and any special problems you may have experienced in the past, such as perms that didn't "take."

Ask for a Hair Analysis Test. A growing number of hair care professionals test the texture, porosity, strength and elasticity of hair with an electronic trichogram or other hair sensing device. That helps to ensure success if you're considering a chemical treatment such as a

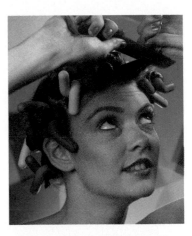

Flexible rubber curlers like these allow you to curl your hair gently, without heat or tugging. They're so comfortable, you even can wear them to bed and get to sleep. While your hair is damp, wind an inch-wide section around each curler, then turn up the ends to secure it in place. Remove the curlers when your hair is dry. (The curlers shown here are Schomy Shapers, available at major department stores.)

Don't Skip the Patch Test

Imagine using a hair-coloring product for years and then applying it one day only to find your neck, face or scalp "dyed"— the skin in those areas red, itchy and swollen. That can— and occasionally does—happen to some people. The reason? Over time, the skin can become allergic to almost any chemical. To prevent this unpleasant surprise, do a patch test *each time* you color your hair. Here's how:

Apply a few drops of the formula to a small area of skin behind one ear and inside an elbow. Leave it on for 24 hours. If any redness, swelling or discomfort results, switch to a different product. (Remember to test the new product, too.)

perm, straightener or coloring. Damaged or weak hair should not be treated until it's back in condition, or it will look ragged and dull.

Find Out about Record Keeping. The best salons keep notes on the dates and types of chemical treatments used on their clients—and the results. That cuts down on guesswork, too.

Observe the Salon's Clients as They Come and Go. Do you like what you see? Good. Or is everyone leaving with carbon-copy hairstyles or outdated cuts? If so, you may be in the wrong place.

Wear Clothes That Express the Personality You Want to Project. If you want a carefree, windblown look, wear jeans or sporty clothes. If you need a conservative, businesslike hairstyle, wear a serious outfit, and so on.

Don't Let Yourself Be Talked into Anything You Don't Want. Granted, we occasionally need to be prodded out of old, boring habits. But unless you're very adventurous or innovative, don't let the stylist talk you into something that sounds too extreme for you. While he or she may be feeling creative, you have to live with the results. By doing your "homework," you control the change, whether it's major or minor.

STYLING AIDS: NEW TWISTS TO OLD STANDBYS

Remember sleeping in curlers? Thanks to a number of time-saving devices and "miracle" setting lotions, no one has to put up with that nonsense anymore (unless they want to).

Curling irons and other electrically heated appliances (see "Hot Rollers: Better Than Ever" on page 44) miraculously curl your hair in just a few minutes, eliminating the need for 8 hours of torture, sleeping in the old wire or plastic curlers.

The miracle, of course, is simple physics plus a pinch of chemistry. Heat alters the molecular structure of hair. It can make straight hair

curly and curly hair straight. There's a tradeoff, though. Heat dries and weakens hair and can damage it in no time unless you take certain precautions.

Also, in addition to "hot" new products, there exists a variety of aids to help those with hair that can't take the heat.

Curling Irons and Hot Combs. To style your hair with a curling iron, grasp each section of hair between the heated tongs. Release after a few seconds and you've got instant curl. To prevent the iron from breaking your hair or burning your scalp, look for a Teflon-coated iron with tiny holes that "steam-set" hair, or "velvet"-coated tongs, and never let the curling iron touch your scalp.

To minimize wear and tear on your tresses, use a curling iron in emergencies or on special occasions, not daily.

Hot combs work on the same principle as curling irons. Used along with a chemical softener, hot combs can straighten kinky or tightly curled hair. But the combination of heat and powerful chemicals can actually dissolve your hair. Ask yourself whether the potential risk is really worthwhile, and consider other ways of styling or relaxing your hair.

Rollers. Brush rollers were designed before anyone realized just how delicate the hair and scalp are. Brush rollers pull, snarl and break hair. Hard, smooth plastic curlers are a bit gentler, provided you don't wind them too tightly.

Soft sponge curlers are the kindest of all to hair and scalp. You can even sleep in them, if you have to. If you're lucky enough to have hair with natural body, you might try this time-saving technique: Roll your hair in sponge curlers before you climb into a hot bath or shower, to let hair steam-set. Afterward, wait until your hair cools and the moist heat has had time to curl your hair. Then unroll your hair, let it air-dry a few minutes and brush gently into place.

Cloth Pincurls and Braids. To set your hair in strips of cotton cloth, twist a section of hair, tie a strip of fabric around the end and roll toward the scalp. Secure the curl by knotting the fabric around the hair nearest the scalp. Unroll and style when dry.

For lots of volume and curl, pincurl your hair. Grasp a section of damp hair, curl it around a finger or two and secure with a hair clip or bobby pin. Let your hair dry, then brush it out.

To add wave to long hair, braid it when it's damp. The fewer and fatter the braids, the looser the waves. Several skinny braids will create crinkly waves. In the meantime, no one will know your hair is "setting." (Be sure not to braid your hair too tightly—the continuous traction will pull hair out of its follicles.)

All of these techniques work best on medium to long hair and take some time. (If you want to speed things up, use the lowest setting on your hair dryer to dry without overdrying.) For short hair, we have still other tricks.

HAIR SPRAYS, MOUSSES AND GELS

Twenty years ago, a television ad for a well-known brand of hair spray showed two young women waterskiing. Their bouffant hairdos survived intact, thanks to hair spray (a mist of water, resin, alcohol and perfume).

In those days, hair spray was so sticky it seemed to glue your hair in place. Nothing short of a hurricane could muss it.

Today's woman is much less intent on cementing every last hair in place. Yet even the most relaxed hairstyles need some "hold." Enter modern hair spray, able to keep hair in place yet so light you can hardly feel it. And today's hair sprays are capable of styling tricks never dreamed of a generation ago, like these two:

- To add volume to short or medium-length hair, lift in sections, spray the roots and "finger comb" the hair as it dries.
- To add volume to long hair, bend over and brush all your hair forward from the nape of the neck. Spray the underside of

the hair and let dry a few seconds. Toss your hair back and style it.

Nonaerosol pump hair sprays work just as well as aerosol sprays and are safer to use. Aerosol products of all kinds disperse a superfine mist of particles that are inhaled into the lungs and quickly absorbed into the bloodstream. Also, one ingredient, the solvent methylene chloride, has caused cancer in animal experiments. Cancer aside, aerosol hair spray can be bothersome to those with asthma or chronic bronchitis or those who are particularly sensitive. These problems are compounded when hair spray is used in small, closed, poorly ventilated spaces. So reach for a pump spray instead.

Mousses and gels are godsends for people with thin, fine or limp hair. Mousse is a foam that looks and feels like shaving cream. Spray some into the palm of your hand, run it through your hair and sculpt waves or peaks or whatever you please. Mousse props hair into place, giving lift where none existed before. (Some mousses add color and conditioners, too, giving you three-dimensional beauty power.)

The new gels (glorified versions of the setting gels of the 1950s and 1960s) work much the same way as mousses. The gels look wet when first applied, then stiffen somewhat as they dry, but when you brush them out, the results are anything but stiff—they give body, volume and lift. Gels can also condition as they style—particularly the ones made with hydrolized human hair keratin protein.

Mousses and gels make short, perky hairstyles possible for people who think their hair is too thin to wear short, or for anyone whose hair needs a little boost. They're ideal for going from pool to party in an hour—or when you don't have the time or inclination to fuss with your hair.

HOW TO HAVE A SAFE PERM

Permanent wave formulas have come a long way since the smelly, frizzy perms some of us had in grade school. They make possible a whole

Five Tips for Longer-Lasting Perms

A perm can look fabulous for the first few days and then fall flat. Here's how to avoid "early letdown."

- Don't shampoo your hair within 48 hours of perming. Shampoo can relax the curl.
- Wait until after your first shampoo to go swimming.
- Use the shampoo and conditioner suggested by your hairdresser. Some over-the-counter products contain compounds such as sodium hydroxide that undo your curls, even after the perm "takes."
- Condition your hair with a product designed specifically for permed hair. That prevents perm "burnout"—dull, dry hair.
- Don't perm your hair more frequently than once every 4 months.

range of natural-looking styles—no matter how fine or limp your hair—without daily curling and fussing.

Even the most expensive perms aren't failsafe, though. How well your perm turns out—and how long it lasts—depends on a number of factors.

Cold waves, which are slightly odorous formulas, soak into the hair shaft, chemically altering the hair. Rolled over rods of various sizes and allowed to set, the hair is then doused with a neutralizing agent to stop the chemical process. Otherwise, the hair would break. As the hair dries, "neutralization" occurs, making the curls permanent.

Heat-activated acid perms work essentially the same way, with an additional step: Heat (from a dryer or heat lamp) helps to set the curls. Heat-activated perms are gentler on your hair but a little tougher on your skin, because heat makes skin more sensitive to strong chemicals of any kind. Dermatologists now say that they treat more people than ever for irritations or allergic reactions to perms. Evidently the combined effect of heat and the perm's active ingredient, glycerol monothioglycolate, can trigger a nasty rash on the face, ears, neck or shoulders.

To sidestep possible reactions, ask your hairdresser to take these precautions:

- Apply a barrier ointment (such as petroleum jelly) around the hairline.
- Wrap absorbent cotton over the barrier.
- Place a thick terrycloth towel around your neck to catch drips.

That's before the solution is applied. Afterward, the hairdresser should do the following:

- Dab away excess perm solution with damp cotton balls.
- Immediately replace the cotton and towel when they become wet. Replace again if necessary.
- Thoroughly rinse the solution from the hair for at least 3 minutes.

If you have very sensitive skin or are prone to skin allergies, ask the salon to do a patch test a week or so ahead of time to see if the solution is safe for you.

Hair that's in good condition takes a perm better than hair that's damaged by weather, hair dryers or coloring. So deep-condition your hair twice a week for a couple of weeks before you perm. And *never* perm and color on the same day—hair can withstand only so much chemical application at one time before it breaks.

Want a sneak preview of how you'd look in curly hair? Try this "one-day" perm. Set your hair on perm rods, spraying each section to be rolled with a mist of water or hair spray. Sit under the dryer for 20 minutes—or let hair air-dry. Then "finger-comb" your hair into loose curls.

What to Do while Your Perm Grows Out

During the last few weeks of a perm's life, hair can begin to develop a dual personality—partly straight, partly wavy. Short of cutting it all off, here are some steps you can take to minimize the contrast between older, wavier hair and newer, straight hair.

- Have your hair trimmed 4 to 6 weeks after the perm. This helps the remaining curl to bounce back to life.
- Use one of the perm revitalizing products on the market, such as Perm Life Perkup by Revlon. They reactivate curl in much the same way that taking a shower will temporarily put spring back into your perm. The difference is that these moisturizing conditioners contain humectants, substances that attract and hold moisture. That helps curls to last longer.
- For short or medium-length perms, add lift by using a styling gel or mousse. Hair care manufacturers are introducing styling products that condition as they style, marketed especially for permed hair.
- If your hair is long and cut in layers, have the ends trimmed and the top spot-permed, to tide you over until the next overall perm.
- If your hair is all one length, ask your stylist to show you how to French-braid your hair. This disguises the difference between new, straight hair and older, wavy hair.

STRAIGHTENERS: "REVERSE PERMS"

People who have naturally curly hair may wish to straighten it, especially if their hair is quite thick or tightly curled. For one thing, tight curls are difficult to style. Straighteners relax the hair to make it easier to comb and style. For another, blacks and other people with tight curls can develop folliculitis, a sort of "acne of the scalp" in which hair follicles become inflamed and sometimes infected. Straighteners alleviate this problem by turning curls away from the scalp and preventing ingrown hairs, which irritate the follicles.

These "reverse perms" may contain sodium hydroxide (lye) or other powerful chemicals that soften the hair. But *over*relaxed hair will break, becoming very short and uneven. Even the milder, lye-free straighteners are caustic enough to burn the skin. So whether you're having your hair straightened professionally or doing it yourself with an over-the-counter product, be careful. Wesley Wilborn, M.D., a dermatologist in Atlanta, Georgia, offers the following advice.

- Test the straightening solution on a small area of the scalp a day or two ahead of time to check for adverse reactions.
- Follow the directions. Never leave the solution on for longer than the manufacturer recommends. And check the hair every few minutes. Straighteners work faster on some people than on others.
- Remove the solution immediately if you feel burning or stinging on your scalp. Don't be afraid to speak up if someone else is applying the solution for you.
- Protect your eyes by wearing a terrycloth sweatband over your forehead and around your neck to catch drips. Handle the solution carefully, so that jerky movements don't splash the solution into your eyes.
- Don't comb or brush wet, freshly straightened hair, especially at the nape of the neck. Wet, treated hair is vulnerable to trauma and may snap off.
- Wait at least two months after your last treatment to have your hair restraightened. Three months would be even better.

In addition, Dr. Wilborn warns people with scalp conditions such as dandruff, seborrhea or psoriasis of the scalp not to use a straightener until the condition clears up. Otherwise, it will get worse.

AN INTELLIGENT PERSON'S GUIDE TO HAIR COLOR

For centuries, people of all ages and both sexes have colored their hair—

Cellophane Dyes: Gentle New Colors

Nervous about trying hair color for the first time? Cellophane (a registered trademark of Sebastian International) could be your best introduction to coloring.

One of the newest and safest hair dyes around, Cellophanes are less apt to irritate skin and eyes than permanent dyes, yet they give comparable, natural-looking results. The Cellophane formula is activated by heat rather than by peroxide or ammonia. The heat opens up the hair cuticle so color can penetrate. By controlling the timing and heat setting, a stylist can control the intensity of color. While Cellophane dyes can't lighten hair, they can darken hair as deeply as you like and they can add highlights to dark hair. They last from 6 to 8 weeks, and they don't run if you perspire or get wet.

Cellophane dyes protect and condition hair as they color, so hair is fuller and more manageable than if you didn't dye it. That's a plus for people with gray hair, which tends to become drier and thinner with age.

Cellophane dyes stain and blend gray fairly well with hair's original color. Browns and golds take best. The stylists we consulted said that Cellophanes are great for anyone who wants to cover gray or enhance basic hair color but doesn't want to take the big step to using a permanent dye. If you're self-conscious about displaying your first gray hairs, Cellophane dyes may be all you need to turn back the clock a couple of years.

and not solely to cover gray. Hair coloring can warm up dull or faded browns, brighten ho-hum blonds, bring out natural reds—or give you a whole new look.

Hair dyes of the past tended to give hair a shoe-polish look. Today, large numbers of natural-looking shades are available. And with few exceptions, they're kind to your hair and scalp. In fact, certain hair-coloring methods—notably henna and semipermanent dyes—actually condition hair and give it body as the product penetrates and swells the hair shaft or coats it like a creme rinse.

Still, colors invariably alter hair structure and chemistry, and each type works differently. To get the most pleasing results, you need to know something about what's available, even if you have your hair professionally colored.

Bleaching. Basically a solution of hydrogen peroxide and other chemicals, hair bleach strips hair of some or all of its pigment—along with lots of moisture. The lighter you want to go, the more bleach you'll require—and the drier your hair will become. After stripping, a toner is usually applied to get the desired shade of blond.

Despite the drying—and possible scalp irritation—bleaching is a very popular means of coloring hair. If you're intent on going blond, look for "gentle lighteners"—mild, permanent, shampoo-in coloring that gives hair a subtly "sun-kissed" look. Lighteners with built-in conditioners are best; they leave hair with a softer feel than bleach alone.

Frosting, tipping and streaking are variations of bleaching that are kinder to your hair than overall bleaching because fewer strands are stripped, minimizing any damage. And selected bleaching reduces the need for monthly touchups.

The key to natural-looking frosting or streaking is the amount of hair you pull through each hole of the frosting cap. (This is a plastic hood with hundreds of tiny holes through which you pull strands of hair with a tool that resembles a crochet hook.) For the more natural, sun-dappled look, pull just a few

strands through the holes. Use more of the holes at the front of the cap, around the face, and less at the back and nape of the neck.

Permanent Dyes. Shampoo-in hair colorings (also called permanent or oxidation-type dyes) are by far the most widely used type of hair color. They contain bleach (to strip hair of natural pigment), peroxide or ammonia (to develop the color) and a number of other ingredients to lock the dye itself into the hair shaft. As with bleaches, the best permanent dyes contain either built-in or follow-up conditioners to buffer the effects of chemicals on hair.

These oxidation-type dyes frequently contain paraphenylenediamine, a chemical that triggers an allergic reaction in approximately 1 out of 100,000 applications. Doing a patch test before every application can forestall a reaction. (See "Don't Skip the Patch Test" on page 46.)

As your hair grows out, you have to reapply permanent dyes to retouch the roots.

Semipermanent Dyes. These penetrate the hair shaft temporarily and last for four to six shampoos. Because they contain neither bleach nor ammonia, semipermanent dyes are milder to the scalp than permanent, oxidation-type dyes. And they rarely trigger allergic reactions.

Semipermanent dyes may appeal to you when you first begin to notice signs of gray, if you've colored your hair before, or if you're not ready to commit yourself to a permanent dye. Gray semipermanent dyes can banish the yellow tones from your gray, making it prettier. Semipermanent dyes can't lighten hair. But they do condition as they color.

Rinses. These don't penetrate the hair shaft at all, so they wash out with every shampoo. Applied to the roots and combed through hair, a rinse can add highlights to your natural color, improve shades of gray or tide you over between permanent color treatments. But the shades may run when you perspire or get wet—a big drawback if you work or play outdoors or pursue sports. And they can rub off on your pillow.

Henna. This vegetable dye—a paste made from henna plants—acts as a stain. Red henna can enhance brown hair with a mahogany sheen. Black henna can darken your natural color. And neutral henna can brighten blond hair, especially when combined with herbs such as camomile or marigold. Because henna does not strip away hair's own pigment, the results depend not so much on the dye as on your individual hair color. It will sufficiently "disguise" hair that is 10 percent or less gray. (That's the earliest stage of graying—if you have large sections of gray, with little or no color showing, you have more than 10 percent.)

To avoid unpredictable results, consult a hair care professional experienced at applying henna. Or use a hair color chart provided by henna distributors.

Henna is probably one of the safest hair-coloring treatments available—it rarely if ever causes an allergic reaction or irritation—and it won't run when wet or shampoo out. As a bonus, henna conditions as it colors because it coats the hair shaft, adding body and shine to dull, lifeless hair. If you have dry hair, add a tablespoon of olive oil or yogurt, or even a whole egg, to the henna paste when mixing it. Remember to always apply it to damp or wet hair. You also can apply henna after a perm, but you can't perm hennaed hair. The perm would lift or change the color.

Metallic, or "Progressive," Dyes. These creams are combed through hair over a period of days. With each application, gray hair becomes progressively darker, until you reach the desired shade.

Most progressive dyes are a dilute solution of lead acetate, deposited on the hair shaft. These deposits can make your hair dry and brittle. Progressive dyes won't respond to conditioners or rub off on clothing and pillows. These dyes also look much more artificial than henna, permanent dyes or semipermanent dyes. And you can't perm your hair or switch to another dye until progressive dye grows out because hair treated with it won't "take" other processes—the coating forms a bar-rier that perms or dyes can't penetrate.

And there's another drawback. Because lead is toxic if absorbed, progressive dyes are potentially harmful. Don't let the dye contact the scalp, and apply with rubber gloves only. Pregnant women should not use these dyes at all.

TROUBLE-FREE HAIR COLOR

No matter what type of dye you decide to use, you'll get the best results if you follow a few basic guidelines.

- Choose a color that's close to your natural color. Going from very light to very dark or very dark to very light is more likely to damage your hair because more chemicals are needed to accomplish the change. And a drastic change—say, from red to coal black—may not harmonize with your skin tones, eye color or eyebrows and lashes.

- Color your hair only if it's in good condition. Healthy hair looks bouncy and shiny. Damaged hair looks limp, dry and dull, with split ends. If your hair has been seriously damaged by perms, bleaches or overdrying, wait until it grows out.

- Do a strand test. Time how long it takes the desired color to develop on one strand before you color your whole head. A strand test shows you how much color to use, how long to leave it on and what it will look like. If you apply color to hair that's already dyed, for instance, you could end up with an entirely different shade than if you apply the same product to untreated hair. Also, permed hair is more porous than unprocessed hair and requires heavier coloring.

- Follow directions. No matter how carefully you've chosen a hair-coloring product, using it incorrectly can undermine the results.

- Use a mild shampoo or one designed especially for color-treated hair. Such a shampoo won't strip color away and cause it to fade.

- Never perm and color on the same day.
- Don't tease, blow-dry or hot-curl bleached hair without applying conditioner.
- Wear a loose-fitting, well-ventilated hat or scarf. This protects color-treated hair from sunlight, heat and perspiration—a combination that can turn hair red or brassy.

There is a question about whether hair dye can cause cancer. A few years ago, some scientific evidence suggested that women who dye their hair increase their risk of developing breast cancer. Closer investigation indicated that women who dye their hair may *not* increase that risk after all, regardless of what kind of dye they use or for how long.

There's still a theoretical possibility that certain hair dyes—such as those containing lead or coal tar—may cause cancer in other parts of the body, since those compounds cause cancer when fed to animals in large amounts.

GETTING RID OF UNWANTED HAIR

In this country, most women routinely shave their legs and underarms, and many include bleaching their "mustaches" in their personal beauty rituals. And with swimsuits cut up high on the leg, hair in the bikini area (the junction of thigh and groin) must also be banished.

People who want to temporarily camouflage or remove superfluous body hair have several options.

Bleaching. Bleaches for facial and body hair (available at drugstores) strip hair of pigment. Dark roots begin to show in a week. Bleaches work better on fair-haired, fair-skinned people than on dark-haired, dark-skinned people. In fact, bleaching can leave permanent light patches on black skin.

Shaving. Quick, simple and inexpensive, shaving is by far the most popular method of removing hair on legs and underarms.

Razors give a closer shave than electric shavers, and hair takes longer to reappear. But no matter which method you choose, any time you shave, you risk irritating your skin. To prevent razor burn or rash, first coat the skin with warm water, soapy lather or a shaving cream or gel. Shave in the direction your hair grows to avoid irritation and in-grown hairs.

Tweezing. This method is reserved mainly for plucking and shaping eyebrows. Use clean, pointy tweezers and a magnifying mirror to help you see what you're doing. To lessen discomfort, place a small plastic bag of ice cubes over your brow for 5 minutes before you begin to tweeze. Don't apply makeup right after tweezing; the open hair follicle can clog and develop a pimple or infection. And never tweeze a hair from a mole or mark on your skin without first consulting a dermatologist.

Chemical Depilatories. These are creams that dissolve hair just below skin level. Depilatories leave a smoother surface than shaving and hair takes longer to grow back.

Depilatories are safer and easier to use than razors for people with raised varicose veins or for diabetics, who must take great care to avoid nicks and cuts.

Anything that's strong enough to dissolve hair can sting or burn the skin, especially if it's left on too long. Depilatories can also permanently lighten or darken black skin. To minimize irritation or potential allergic reactions, buy products designed specifically for the legs, face or bikini area. Some contain soothing ingredients to buffer harsh chemicals and reduce irritation.

Read and follow the directions. Most manufacturers recommend that you test the lotion on a small, inconspicuous area—such as the inside of your arm at the elbow—for 10 minutes or so. If no redness or irritation occurs within 24 hours, the depilatory is probably safe for you to use.

Waxing. To wax off hair, melt a chunk of depilatory wax, cool it to a comfortable, tepid temperature and stroke it on your skin in the direction hair grows, working on a small section at a time. When the wax hardens, strip it off in the opposite direction. Hair trapped in the wax is pulled out from the root—much like tweezing. Cold wax formulas can be applied at room temperature. These products often include disposable cloth strips: The strip is pressed into the wax, and when the wax hardens you can peel it off in one quick, easy motion.

Waxing lasts longer than shaving or depilatories, but it has drawbacks. Mild discomfort is one of them. Removing the wax feels like pulling adhesive tape off your skin. And you can't wax again until about ¼ inch of hair grows back.

People who want to keep their legs smooth all the time would be better off with frequent shaving or depilatories. Also, infections, small tears in the skin and inflammation are common after waxing. You can minimize those risks by dusting your skin with powder or smoothing on mineral oil before applying wax.

ELECTROLYSIS: HIGH-TECH HAIR REMOVAL

If you have little patience with temporary hair removal methods, electrolysis may be for you. Basically, a fine needle (either straight or bulbous) is inserted into the hair follicle. A mild electrical charge zaps each hair at its root, and the dead hairs are lifted out once and for all. Electrolysis is a long-term process and it's not without possible discomfort. But it is the only permanent method of hair removal—and that's a big advantage.

"Electrolysis is now viewed the way the use of hair dyes was 40 years ago—people are having it done but not telling," says Katherine Heaviside, spokesperson for the International Guild of Professional Electrologists.

If you should experience discomfort during electrolysis, try applying ice packs before and after each session. For an extremely sensitive area, such as the upper lip, Ms. Heaviside suggests you ask your dentist to give you a shot of Novocaine beforehand. (Other areas have fewer

nerve endings and do not require any kind of anesthetic.)

Expect to have several 15-minute appointments, depending on how much hair needs to be removed. The initial sessions may catch only the 85 percent or so of hair that's in the growth stage. Dormant hair may not surface until weeks or months later, calling for an occasional follow-up session. And coarser hairs are more difficult to remove, because the roots are larger or may not be completely destroyed in one attempt. Electrolysis may trigger keloids (thick scars), to which blacks are particularly susceptible. So, if you're black, waxing or shaving may be better choices.

Electrolysis is only as good as the electrologist who does it. Too much current can scar the skin. So don't use a home electrolysis kit. Instead, find a competent, well-trained professional electrologist. Write to the International Guild of Professional Electrologists, Medical Center, 15 Bond Street, Great Neck, NY 10021 for the names of certified (and, in some states, licensed) electrologists in your area. Enclose a stamped, self-addressed envelope.

Electrolysis: A First-Hand Report

What's electrolysis really like? Does it hurt? One woman who tried it to defuzz her upper lip shared her experience with us.

"Chemical hair removers irritated my face terribly and had to be reapplied too often, so I finally tried electrolysis. I wouldn't say it was painful—I felt a tingling sensation while the roots were zapped. The area right underneath my nose was the most sensitive, but I grew accustomed to the feeling as the treatments progressed. The process took several 15-minute sessions, totaling about 4 hours.

"My skin looked a little red after each session, like a mild sunburn. I applied a cool soothing lotion and by the time I returned to work, the redness disappeared.

"Electrolysis left no scars whatsoever. I go back to the electrologist once every 5 or 6 months to have a solitary hair or two removed. But it's nothing compared to the hundreds of hairs I started out with.

"I would recommend electrolysis to anyone needlessly bothered by unwanted hair growth."

Trouble-Free Hair: Easy Solutions to Tough Problems

Hair can be fickle. For a while, your hair will look terrific. Then one morning, without warning, your locks lose their bounce. Or explode into frizz. Or ooze more oil than a Saudi well. Turn to this troubleshooting guide to solve stubborn or unexpected hair trouble.

Dull Hair

POSSIBLE CAUSES

Soapy residue
Damage from sun, overdrying, chemical treatments

WHAT TO DO

Rinse thoroughly with weak solution of white vinegar in water (2 tablespoons to a quart of water) after every shampoo
Use an instant conditioner after every shampoo and deep-condition weekly

Fine or Limp Hair

POSSIBLE CAUSES

Heredity (small hair follicles)
Using incorrect conditioner (for example, a conditioner for dry, damaged hair will overcondition normal or oily hair)
Inadequate rinsing of shampoo or conditioner (or both)

WHAT TO DO

Short, blunt cut adds body
Body wave or perm will add volume, hide scalp and disguise the problem
Use conditioner, mousse or gel
Fine hair may need conditioner on the ends *only*

Flyaway Hair

POSSIBLE CAUSE

Static electricity plus dryness

WHAT TO DO

Use a creme rinse to reverse the electrical charge on hair shaft

Dry Hair

POSSIBLE CAUSES

Heredity (oil glands do not produce enough oil to lubricate hair shaft)
Overuse or improper use of heat appliances (dryers, curling irons, hot rollers)
Chemical treatments (perms, straighteners, bleaches)
Chlorinated pool water
Frequent exposure to sun and wind

WHAT TO DO

Use a shampoo and conditioner formulated for dry hair
Let dry naturally, or blow-dry on low, cool setting. Stop blow-drying before hair is completely dry
Deep-condition weekly
Wear a rubber cap when swimming
Condition after swimming
Wear a hat or scarf outdoors

Thinning Hair

POSSIBLE CAUSES

Hormonal changes due to pregnancy, childbirth, menopause, aging and various metabolic conditions
Emotional stress
Improper diet

WHAT TO DO

Comb, brush, set very gently
Use a conditioner to thicken hair shafts
Cut and style to maximize volume
Be sure you are getting at least 10 milligrams (for men) or 18 milligrams (for women) of iron a day and 46 grams (for men) or 56 grams (for women) of protein a day
See a doctor to check other, hard-to-identify causes

Frizzies

POSSIBLE CAUSE

Effect of humidity on curly or
porous hair (overprocessed by
perms, coloring, overexposure
to sun and wind)

WHAT TO DO

Cut off damaged hair; have hair
cut all one length, not layered

Don't perm hair immediately before
hot, humid season (summer, in
most places)

Use a creme rinse after every
shampoo

If hair is short, blow-dry gently,
smoothing hair as it dries

If hair is medium-length or long,
roll to straighten and smooth
frizz

Tangles

POSSIBLE CAUSES

Hair shafts roughened by razor
cuts, chemical treatments,
"teasing," other damage

WHAT TO DO

Scissor cut only

After shampoo, pat hair dry; don't
tousle

Use a creme rinse after every
shampoo to "polish" hair and
prevent tangles

Gently coax out tangles with
fingers, then with wide-toothed
comb

Dandruff

POSSIBLE CAUSES

Scalp bacteria

Hormone production

Oil gland malfunction

Infrequent shampoos

Improper rinsing

Overconditioning

Sunburned scalp

WHAT TO DO

Shampoo frequently

Rinse thoroughly

Dab scalp with cotton balls soaked
with a dilute solution of 1 part
witch hazel or lemon juice to 4
parts water

Use a dandruff shampoo

Wear a hat or scarf outdoors

Split Ends

POSSIBLE CAUSES

Dry, brittle hair

Setting hair in brush rollers

Chlorinated pool water

Rough treatment: Too-vigorous
towel-drying, overdrying, brushing too hard or too often or
with a brush with ragged, rough-
edged bristles, tugging at
tangles, back-combing or
"teasing"

WHAT TO DO

Cut off split ends, a little at a
time if they reach the scalp

Condition hair after every shampoo to minimize visible damage
and prevent further splitting

Use soft, smooth rollers

Wear rubber cap when swimming

Never brush hair when wet. Ease
out tangles gently with a wide-
toothed comb

Do not backcomb or "tease" hair

Greenish Hair

POSSIBLE CAUSE

Discoloring effect of algicides
(algae-control chemicals) added
to chlorinated pool water. Usually affects blond hair, especially very light blond hair

WHAT TO DO

Wear a rubber cap when swimming and/or apply a conditioner
afterward

Rinse with fresh water as soon as
possible after swimming

Shampoo with Ultraswim or other
antichlorine shampoo

Rinse with camomile tea every
other week to restore blondness

Oily Hair

POSSIBLE CAUSES

Heredity (oil glands produce more
oil than necessary)

Infrequent shampoos

Use of conditioner containing too
much oil

WHAT TO DO

Buy a shampoo and conditioner
formulated for oily hair

Wash hair, rinse, wash again, leaving shampoo on scalp for 5 minutes before final, thorough rinse

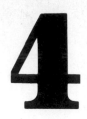

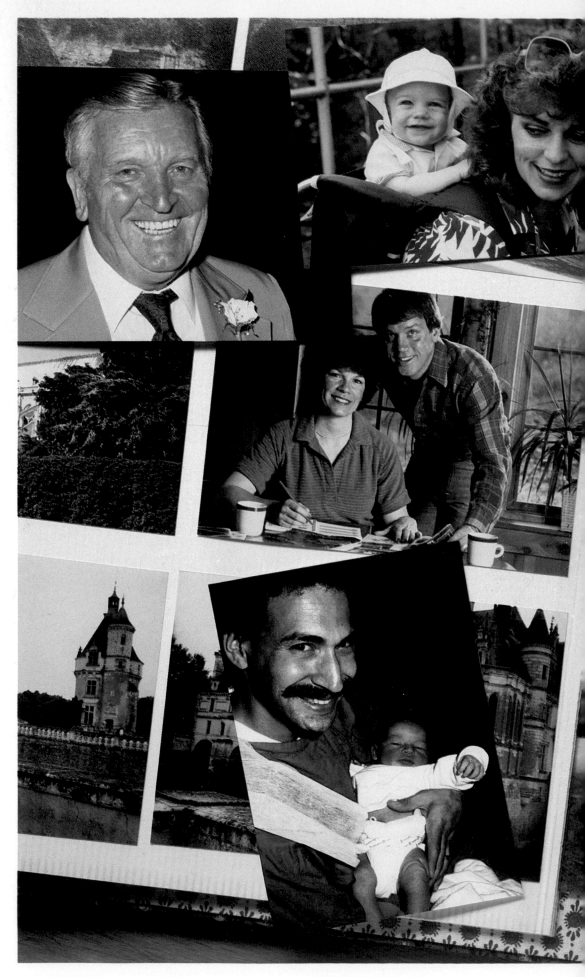

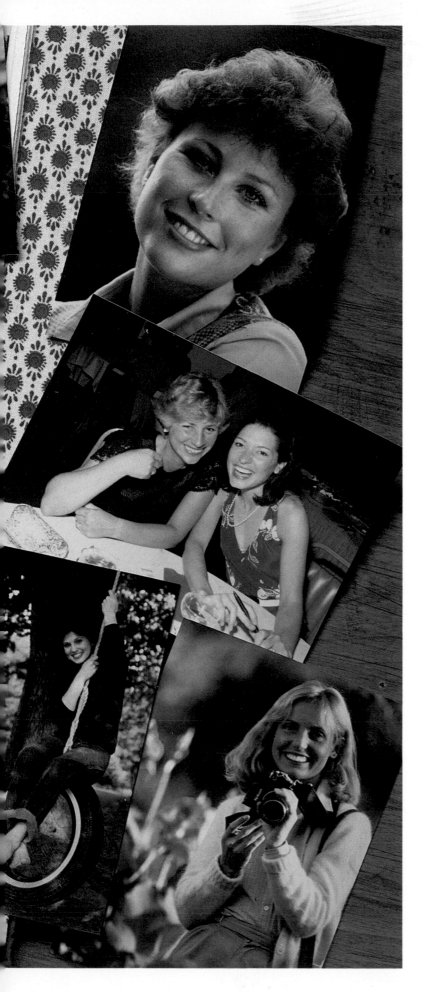

The Smile Factor

Here's a beauty program to give anyone terrific teeth.

Your mouth communicates—even when you're silent. The sullen line of disappointment. The full, open smile of joy. All these and countless other emotions are revealed without speech. But your mouth also reveals a lot about your health.

Your lips are a sensitive barometer of your body's internal states. When you're cold, your lips turn blue. When you're dehydrated, your lips are, too. Certain nutritional deficiencies show up as changes in the lips, teeth and gums before they show up on a lab report.

Your teeth are an indispensable part of the scaffolding that supports your lips and cheeks. Changes in your teeth and jaw that commonly occur with age can alter the shape of the face, making you look older—maybe even less healthy—than you really are.

Because your mouth is your most mobile facial feature, it serves as the centerpiece of your facial expression. A winning smile is both a physical and a psychological asset. If you have one, you'll feel better about yourself and others will respond positively to you. A confident, gleaming smile can transform even lackluster, nondescript features into a warm, inviting, attractive face. And whether you smile or pout, moist, color-tinged lips are sexy. So are strong, blemish-free teeth.

Smile at the nearest magnifying mirror. What do you see? Smooth, soft lips? Even, white teeth? Firm, pink gums that hug each tooth securely? Or does your smile make you self-conscious, make you appear older than you really are?

Whatever shape your smile is in—even if it makes you frown—there are easy, effective ways to restore (or maintain) its beauty and radiance. Where do you begin? Not surprisingly, with the teeth.

THE ART AND SCIENCE
OF BEAUTIFUL TEETH

When you think of Chinese inventions, you probably think of gunpowder and silk. Well, they pale in significance next to China's major accomplishment, the toothbrush. And you'll lose face unless you honor Chinese ingenuity: To keep your smile youthful, you have to brush regularly.

But proper brushing means more than a quick go-round with any old toothbrush. Dentists almost universally recommend a soft nylon brush with round-tipped bristles and a flat brushing surface. The head should be small enough to reach all your teeth, even if you have to use a child-sized toothbrush.

Hold the toothbrush sideways with the bristles at a 45-degree angle to your teeth, so that they can slip under the flap of gum that hugs each tooth. Move the brush back and forth in short, semicircular motions. Make sure to brush the front, inner and outer surfaces of your teeth.

To brush the back of your upper and lower front teeth, hold the brush vertically and brush up and down with short strokes. For the chewing surfaces, scrub back and forth gently with short strokes.

If your gums bleed easily when you brush, don't brush less in the belief that they need lighter treatment. Brush *more*. Bleeding results from the accumulation of plaque, the soft, sticky coating of food and bacteria that clings to teeth and gums the way barnacles cling to seaside rocks. At the very least, fermenting plaque will mar your teeth and sour your breath. At the worst, plaque will contribute to tooth loss.

Plaque is the first sign of periodontal disease (inflamed or infected gums), but it is reversible. Gum disease causes more adult tooth loss than tooth decay. Plaque and tartar (its hardened state) cause gums to swell or recede and can cause straight teeth to drift and wobble. Plaque can also form pockets in the gums that give sanctuary to further debris and decay-causing bacteria. If plaque-induced gum disease gets out of hand, you might have to undergo gum surgery—a painful, time-consuming and expensive treatment. So while you may have left behind the so-called cavity-prone years, your

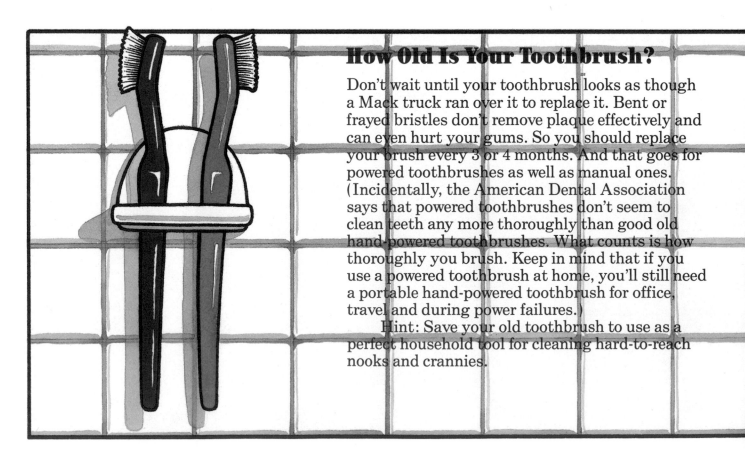

How Old Is Your Toothbrush?

Don't wait until your toothbrush looks as though a Mack truck ran over it to replace it. Bent or frayed bristles don't remove plaque effectively and can even hurt your gums. So you should replace your brush every 3 or 4 months. And that goes for powered toothbrushes as well as manual ones. (Incidentally, the American Dental Association says that powered toothbrushes don't seem to clean teeth any more thoroughly than good old hand-powered toothbrushes. What counts is how thoroughly you brush. Keep in mind that if you use a powered toothbrush at home, you'll still need a portable hand-powered toothbrush for office, travel and during power failures.)

Hint: Save your old toothbrush to use as a perfect household tool for cleaning hard-to-reach nooks and crannies.

teeth and gums need as much care now as ever. Don't slack off.

WHICH TOOTHPASTE IS BEST FOR YOU?

Choosing a toothpaste is much like choosing a shampoo. How do you separate hype from fact?

All toothpastes are abrasive. That's their main source of cleaning power. The best dentifrice is one that is abrasive enough to prevent stains and plaque buildup yet not harsh enough to injure teeth or gums, says a representative of the American Dental Association (ADA). Dental enamel can resist some abrasion, but don't overdo it.

If you need only a slight degree of abrasion to clean teeth of stains, you can use baking soda, says the ADA. Other people may need a commercial toothpaste, which may contain any of a number of abrasive mineral compounds, such as dicalcium phosphate or dehydrated silica gel. Smokers, for example, usually need the added cleaning power of a com-mercial toothpaste. Don't brush too vigorously or too frequently, or you'll gradually wear down the tooth enamel.

Commercial toothpastes have one definite edge over plain baking soda: Many contain fluoride, a mineral that is incorporated into tooth enamel and helps to prevent tooth decay *throughout life*. Fluoride toothpastes that display the seal of the American Dental Association's Council on Dental Therapeutics are effective against tooth decay.

Another potential advantage of commercial toothpaste is that it makes brushing more pleasant, prompting you to brush regularly. Commercial toothpastes contain foaming agents, such as sodium lauryl sulfate, that feel good in your mouth. Humectants such as glycerol keep toothpaste from drying out should someone leave the cap off the tube (a heinous crime in most households). Flavoring helps to give each brand its special appeal.

We should mention that stubborn smoking stains also point to a more serious problem. Smoking may speed up osteoporosis, a common

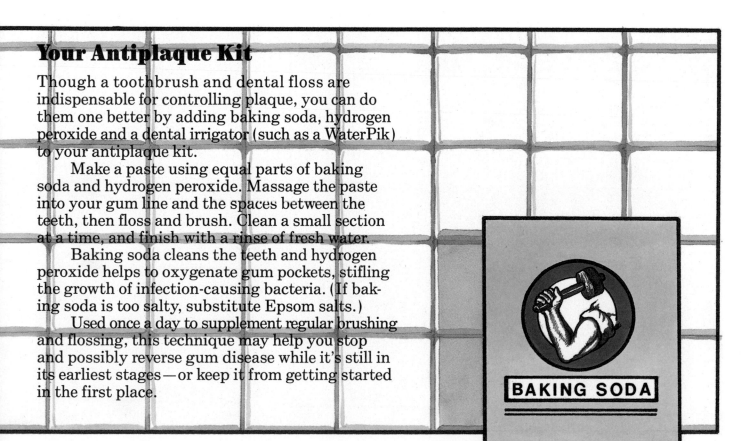

Your Antiplaque Kit

Though a toothbrush and dental floss are indispensable for controlling plaque, you can do them one better by adding baking soda, hydrogen peroxide and a dental irrigator (such as a WaterPik) to your antiplaque kit.

Make a paste using equal parts of baking soda and hydrogen peroxide. Massage the paste into your gum line and the spaces between the teeth, then floss and brush. Clean a small section at a time, and finish with a rinse of fresh water.

Baking soda cleans the teeth and hydrogen peroxide helps to oxygenate gum pockets, stifling the growth of infection-causing bacteria. (If baking soda is too salty, substitute Epsom salts.)

Used once a day to supplement regular brushing and flossing, this technique may help you stop and possibly reverse gum disease while it's still in its earliest stages—or keep it from getting started in the first place.

BAKING SODA

condition (particularly among women) in which bones (including the jawbone) grow porous and brittle. As a result, women with osteoporosis are *three times* as likely to lose all their teeth before age 60 as women without osteoporosis, according to a study in *Archives in Internal Medicine.* Makes one wonder about those glamorous ads showing liberated women puffing their favorite brand of cigarette.

HOW TO FLOSS WITHOUT GETTING FLUSTERED

No toothbrush or dentifrice can reach the tight spaces between teeth that make perfect hideouts for plaque. That's where dental floss comes in. Nothing works quite like floss to dislodge plaque. Here's how to use it to its best advantage.

Break off a piece of floss about 18 inches long. Tie the ends together in a double knot to form a loop that's easy to manage. Grasp a portion of floss about 1½ inches long between the thumb and forefinger of each hand. Holding the floss taut, gently slide it between your upper front teeth (since they're the easiest to reach).

Curve the floss into a C-shape around one tooth, easing the string into the space between the gum and tooth until you feel some resistance. Hold the floss snugly against the tooth and slide it up and down along the side of the tooth, using a sawing motion.

Curve the floss around the adjacent tooth and repeat. Use a fresh portion of floss for each tooth, wiping accumulated saliva and plaque onto a tissue, then winding the used portion of floss around your left forefinger. You'll probably need a second loop of floss by the time you get to your lower teeth.

After you've flossed all your teeth, rinse your mouth with water to wash away any loosened plaque.

Flossing takes some getting used to. Your first attempt may take 15 minutes and seem messy or awkward. Don't worry if your gums bleed the first two or three times you floss—that's normal. Soon the bleeding will stop and flossing will take only 5 minutes.

Dentists we consulted said that whether you use waxed or unwaxed floss isn't terribly important; they're equally effective. Just be sure to floss *daily,* without fail. Plaque forms constantly, day or night, whether or not you eat. Dislodging plaque by brushing thoroughly and flossing once a day interrupts plaque formation and prevents it from destroying your teeth and gums.

You might want to floss at night to interrupt plaque formation while you sleep. If you can floss at night, great. But if you're one of those people who don't feel like doing much more than brushing their teeth and tumbling into bed at night, chances are you'll be more conscientious about flossing if you couple it with a morning ritual, such as applying your makeup or shaving.

THE CLEANING PROS

You probably never thought of your dentist or dental hygienist as a beauty consultant, but both are indispensable to people who want attractive smiles. Professional clean-

---

Check Your Teeth for Plaque

The trouble with plaque is that you can't see the damage it does to your gums until it's too late. Dentists, fortunately, came up with "disclosing" tablets and liquids—products that temporarily stain plaque so you can see any buildup. You can buy disclosing dye at the drugstore to monitor plaque yourself and tell if you're thoroughly cleaning your teeth.

Swish the liquid around in your mouth or chew the tablets before and after you floss and brush. Repeat this process every day for a week or so. (Be careful not to swallow the dye or splash any on your clothes.) Stained areas on your teeth indicate spots where you need to floss and brush more carefully. After the first week, with careful cleaning, you shouldn't have to use disclosing dye more than once a week or so, to spot-check for plaque.

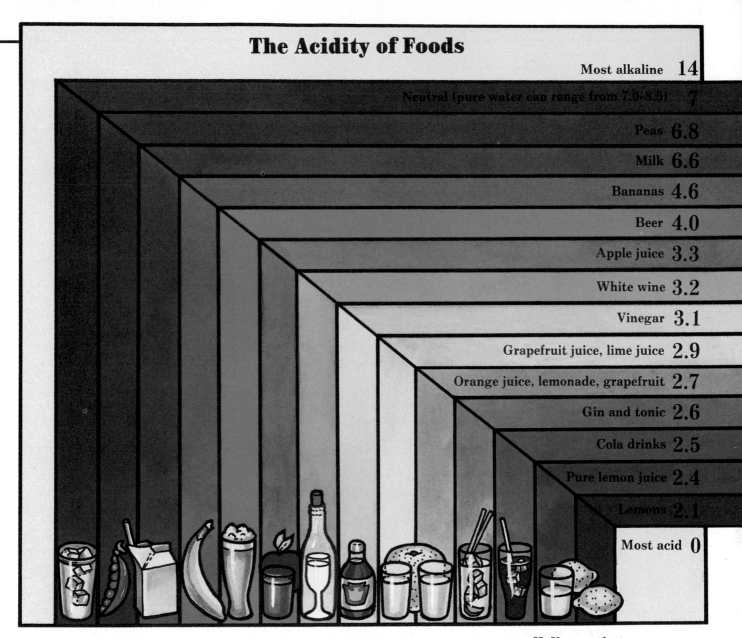

The Acidity of Foods

Most alkaline	**14**
Neutral (pure water can range from 7.0-8.5)	**7**
Peas	**6.8**
Milk	**6.6**
Bananas	**4.6**
Beer	**4.0**
Apple juice	**3.3**
White wine	**3.2**
Vinegar	**3.1**
Grapefruit juice, lime juice	**2.9**
Orange juice, lemonade, grapefruit	**2.7**
Gin and tonic	**2.6**
Cola drinks	**2.5**
Pure lemon juice	**2.4**
Lemons	**2.1**
Most acid	**0**

ing reaches places you can't, removing plaque and stains that develop no matter how conscientiously you brush and floss. (After all, even a dentist goes to the dentist.)

While most dentists recommend going for professional cleanings every six months or so, individual needs can vary. People who smoke or drink a lot of coffee or tea, for example, will need to have their teeth professionally cleaned more frequently than those who don't. On the other hand, if your teeth show no stains or tartar formation, you may not need to have your teeth cleaned as frequently.

Cleaning techniques are better than ever, thanks to modern dental technology. In addition to routine scaling and polishing, your dentist may have a number of techniques and gadgets to tackle the most stubborn stains and deposits.

One is an instrument called a Prophy Jet. The size of a large marking pen, this tool delivers to the tooth surface a high-speed stream of air, warm water and a special form of sodium bicarbonate. The solution dissolves stubborn stains in seconds, without wearing down tooth enamel.

Another innovative device is an ultrasonic scaler, which vibrates at about 20,000 cycles per second. The vibrating tip breaks up plaque deposits the way a jackhammer breaks up street pavement—only much more quietly and gently. The result is cleaner, healthier teeth and gums.

For the cavity-prone, one dentist we spoke to bathes teeth in a solution containing very small amounts of iodine and iodide, which wipes out germs (*Streptococcus*

pH. You see the term on shampoos: A low pH is acid, high is alkaline. Well, the Swiss also mark their *food* with labels based on the pH, maybe because their addiction to neatness and cleanliness extends to their teeth. Foods with a low or acid pH can pit and discolor teeth. So how can you eat those foods (many of which are loaded with nutrients) and still have a smile that's legal in Switzerland?

After you eat acidic foods (see the list above), rinse your mouth with water. Or you can add a bit of baking soda to the water; it's alkaline and may help neutralize the acid. And if you brush your teeth after the meal, wait at least 20 minutes; teeth are more vulnerable to abrasion immediately after you eat acid foods.

mutans) that cause cavities. The rinse decimates the entire population of bacteria immediately. What's more, the germs take four to six months to regroup and flourish.

Good-looking, healthy teeth depend 90 percent on self-care and 10 percent on professional care. Regular checkups catch microscopic problems, like pinhole cavities and slight gum recession, before they grow into big, ugly problems. In that way, regular checkups serve as preventive maintenance for your smile.

WHAT'S EATING YOUR TEETH?

Lustrous, pearly, stain-free teeth look terrific on anyone. Should your pearls discolor—or worse yet, become pitted and gritty—something's amiss. Chances are, acid of some kind is to blame. Your teeth can take only so much.

One woman, for example, was distraught to discover that her teeth were rough and pitted after an all-night tequila-drinking bout. Following custom, she had chased each shot of tequila by sucking on a lime wedge—one of nature's most concentrated sources of acid. (See "The Acidity of Foods" on page 61.)

Acids of all kinds are notorious "etchers," and citrus fruit and other acid foods, if used in excess, can actually leach calcium out of the tightly packed crystals that form tooth enamel.

Smooth, pearly teeth may turn rough, dull gray or yellow because the loss of their white enamel coating exposes underlying dentin, which is darker and duller than enamel. Dentin stains easily and is harder to scrub clean than enamel, too. And plaque adheres more readily to a rough surface than to a smooth one.

You don't necessarily have to quaff tequila and lime to discolor your teeth, though. Cola drinks, vinegar, apple juice, beer and wine are also acidic. Sugar of any kind fosters *Streptococcus mutans.* In the process of devouring your mouth's sugars, this bacteria produces enamel-dissolving acid.

The extent of the resulting damage depends on how much sugary and/or acidic food you consume and how often you consume it. Your teeth are probably safe if, for example, you drink orange juice with breakfast, a soda in the afternoon and a glass of wine with dinner. But if you sip one soda after another during the course of the day, or routinely polish off a six-pack of beer every night, steady contact with acids could slowly eat away your teeth, leaving them scratchy and dull. British doctors have noticed that people who habitually sip warm lemon juice—an old English folk remedy—to soothe a cold or sore throat often develop pitted teeth.

Because a certain amount of enamel erosion occurs naturally over the years, avoiding overexposure to acids becomes especially important as you grow older. Drinking fruit juice, soft drinks and other beverages through a straw shunts the acid away from your teeth and minimizes its effect. So does rinsing your mouth with water, which is neutral (neither acid nor alkaline).

Chewing on aspirin or vitamin C tablets can also erode teeth. So can chewing on hydrochloric acid tablets, a digestive aid. Swallow these pills without chewing them, even if you have to break them first.

DENTAL RENEWALS

Say your teeth are already pitted. Or deeply stained. Or crooked. Or

---

Braces: Not Just Kid Stuff

Do you ever wish you'd had an opportunity to have your teeth straightened earlier in life? Now that you're older, there's still hope for a perfect bite. (Straight teeth are healthy teeth at any age.) What's more, adult bites aren't any more difficult to correct than those of teenagers—in fact, braces sometimes work *faster* on grownups, who tend to be more cooperative.

Nowadays dentists apply about 1 out of 6 sets of braces to adult teeth. If you'd feel self-conscious about flashing so much metal when you smile or speak, ask about clear plastic, "invisible" braces, worn behind the teeth, or removable braces that you can wear only at night.

missing. Don't despair. Almost no dental problem is beyond salvage (see "Cosmetic Dentistry: What It Can Correct"). Dentistry can patch, anchor, realign and replace teeth so you don't have to live with a conspicuous problem. A very small improvement in your teeth can make an enormous difference in your overall appearance—and your health.

Orthodontics. Don't feel vain about wanting to have your teeth straightened, even if only one or two teeth are slightly crooked. Straighter teeth are healthier teeth, because crooked or crowded teeth are difficult to clean and provide hiding places for plaque and bacteria. Protruding teeth can force you to breathe through your mouth instead of your nose, irritating and inflaming your gums and leading to more frequent colds, coughs and sore throats, since the nose doesn't get a chance to moisturize, filter and purify air before it reaches the upper respiratory tract. An improper bite can also prevent you from enjoying chewy, fibrous foods, contributing to constipation and other possible digestive problems. And misaligned teeth can even cause headaches and facial pain.

Bonding. Coating teeth with a composite resin covers stains and discolorations. Bonding can also fill decayed teeth, replace large, unsightly gold or silver fillings and close unsightly spaces or gaps—all at a fraction of the time and cost of more elaborate procedures such as braces or crowns.

In bonding, the dentist first etches the tooth with a mild acid gel, then applies an enamel-dentin bonding agent. Using special tools, the dentist then hand-sculpts the resin veneer, a puttylike material made of plastic and finely ground glass, to provide a natural, translucent surface that hardens and looks no different from other healthy teeth nearby. A skilled, artistic dentist can apply the veneer in thin layers, blending various shades together to achieve a completely natural appearance.

Bonding is a godsend to people whose teeth are permanently stained because they took tetracycline as children, before doctors realized that

the antibiotic could stain developing teeth. As teens, their teeth developed a definite gray color. The effects appear around the time teens enter junior high school—just when youngsters become most self-conscious about their appearance. Needless to say, bonding can provide a tremendous boost to self-image.

"You really can see someone's personality change," says Terry F. Crawford, D.D.S., associate professor of operative dentistry at Emory University in Atlanta, Georgia. "After several weeks, sometimes even after just one visit, they show more confidence, a better self-image. The teenager who never smiled in class pictures or who always held his or her hand over their mouth no longer feels like an outcast."

Dentists can also use bonding to seal off cavities—a welcome alternative if you dislike having your teeth drilled (and who doesn't?). When the dentist finds a small cavity, he or she paints the affected tooth with composite resin, which shields the cavity from decay-causing bacteria and stops it from getting any bigger. This technique is especially useful for containing tiny cavities in the microscopic grooves in the back teeth.

Bonding is an art, requiring meticulous skill and lots of practice. The more experienced your dentist, the better you'll look. Don't be afraid to ask to see "before and after" pictures of any other bonding work done by the dentist you are considering. If the dentist has pride in the workmanship, you will, too. Also, you deserve an attentive consultation. Being ushered in and out of the office in 5 minutes suggests that the dentist may not take great care to get your teeth just right.

Crowns. Sometimes called caps, crowns can also repair stained, chipped or misshapen teeth, especially if the problem is more than superficial. Crowns can also save badly decayed or crumbling teeth. And they can salvage loose teeth by forming a splint with nearby tighter teeth, thereby extending the life of natural teeth for many years despite existing gum disease.

Crowns can also improve your

profile. If, for example, you have a substantial underbite so that your lower lip juts forward in a continual pout, crowns can build up the upper teeth to equalize your smile.

To fashion a crown, the dentist grinds your own tooth down to a stump (while your mouth is anesthetized) and fits a jacket of porcelain, gold or other material over it. The best crowns are made of procelain (which is beautiful) fused to gold (which is strong). Crowns may also be made of plastic or stainless steel, or combinations of materials. A crown looks and functions like your own tooth—or better. Crowns are more expensive and require more work than bonding, but they last longer.

BRIDGING THE GAP

Most adults in this country lose at least one tooth after age 30 and even more after age 40. Sometimes the loss results from poor oral hygiene and sometimes from occurrences like auto accidents or sports mishaps (this is especially true for young adults.)

While most people wouldn't hesitate to replace a missing front tooth, many feel that one less back tooth makes no difference in health or appearance. That's not so. For one thing, a missing tooth can prompt remaining teeth to shift, which can eventually lead to loss of more teeth. Even worse, as the years pass, your cheeks will cave in toward the empty spaces left by missing teeth, causing your face to sag, pucker and wrinkle like a deflated balloon.

Fixed bridgework is probably a good way to prevent this kind of premature aging. As the term suggests, fixed bridgework functions much like a bridge spanning a gorge: Artificial teeth are attached to crowns anchored over good teeth on each side of the gap left by missing teeth.

Once bridgework is in place, you won't be able to tell your artificial teeth from your natural teeth— they'll look and perform just as well. Fixed bridgework costs more than partial dentures (removable plates) because of the more elaborate engineering involved. But bridgework is far better for your health and appearance than dentures. With a partial denture, the metal clasps that hold the plate in place are a dead give-away that you wear "false teeth." The clasps also trap food particles and can hasten the decay of your real teeth. Food also tends to collect under the plate and may cause bad breath, no matter how carefully you try to clean it. And a partial denture is a foreign object in your mouth, so it may interfere with speech, feel uncomfortable and slip out.

Fixed bridgework, on the other hand, defies detection. One woman we know was married for two years before she found out that her husband's front teeth were a bridge. And that's only because her mother-in-law accidentally revealed the information.

No matter what type of restoration you decide on—bonding, crowns or bridgework—you want it to look convincing. Since adult teeth just aren't as white as they were at age 14, no matter how well they're cared for, don't be disappointed when the dentist matches the color of your new teeth to your old ones. Pure white teeth would look phony and announce to the world that you're wearing false teeth. The same is true for alignment: Too-perfect teeth look too good to be true; *slight* irregularities are more convincing.

Lastly, there is the option of full dentures. Never let anyone talk you into having your natural teeth replaced with dentures until you've exhausted every possible method of retaining them. Full dentures eventually settle, aging your facial appearance unnecessarily. And they're very uncomfortable.

If dentures *are* your only alternative, buy the best you can afford. Before you accept the dentures, use the following criteria to determine whether they look right.

- Do your lips and cheeks drape aesthetically?
- How much gum shows when you smile?
- Does the vertical midline of the dentures line up with the tip of your nose?
- Are the shape and shade of the teeth flattering—not artificially white or straight?

Twelve Ways to Lick Dry Lips

Licking chapped lips only makes them worse. Here are a dozen better alternatives to soothe dry, sore lips:

All-Purpose Basics
Lanolin
Mineral oil
Petroleum jelly
Vegetable oil
Vitamin A
Vitamin E

Lip Care Products
ChapStick
Lip gloss
Lip smoothers
Moisturizing
  lipstick
Vaseline Constant
  Care
Vaseline Lip
  Therapy

CAN YOU AFFORD COSMETIC DENTISTRY?

The types of cosmetic dentistry we've been talking about aren't just for movie stars or wealthy folks. Melvin Denholtz, D.D.S., chief of dental research at Newark Beth Israel Hospital in New Jersey, puts it this way: "You can probably have your chipped front tooth repaired with a composite resin for less than the price of dinner for two. You can probably have several teeth capped for no more than you spent on your last vacation. Even getting your buck teeth straightened . . . can cost you less than your monthly car payments."

Considering the return on your investment in terms of health and self-image, cosmetic dentistry is money well spent.

Take the case of Bernard, age 47. His periodontist told him he had advanced gum disease. Bernard had two choices: The doctor could restore his gums, correct his bite and crown his teeth—admittedly a sizable investment in time and money. The alternative was to extract all of Bernard's teeth and fit him for full dentures. To Bernard, losing all his teeth meant loss of virility, sex appeal and youthfulness. So he chose option one, the dental "facelift."

Sometimes, even people who can easily afford dental work feel guilty or self-conscious about the possibility of bonding, crowns or braces. They needn't.

"Cosmetic dentistry done to erase a mistake of nature or to retard the aging process should *not* lay a guilt trip on you," says Dr. Denholtz. "If it is within your means, why not enjoy it?"

Fixing your teeth may also improve your lips. Because lips are supported by a scaffolding of teeth, straightening or otherwise repositioning teeth can make lips wider or narrower, thicker or thinner, more or less prominent—often for the better.

LIPS WORTH SMILING ABOUT

Picture the Mona Lisa with chapped lips. Ruins the effect, right? Don't

let dry, chapped lips ruin your smile.

Your first instinct will be to lick chapped lips. Don't. Licking your lips only makes matters worse. Cold wintry air or arid summer breezes evaporate moisture and lead to further irritation, peeling and sometimes bleeding.

The only way to solve the problem is to create a protective barrier between your lips and dry air with a moisturizing oil or cream of some type. You can choose from hundreds of products (see "Twelve Ways to Lick Dry Lips"). Even lipstick can act as a moisturizer. Wearing a very thin film of petroleum jelly or baby oil underneath your lipstick can double your protection. (Let it soak in for a minute or two before applying lipstick, so lip color will adhere better.)

Apply the oily barrier before and after you go outdoors, or frequently if you work in a dry indoor environment. It's a good idea to give your lips an occasional exposure to dry air, though. Otherwise they become dependent on moisturizers and "forget" how to adapt to the environment when you stop using lip balm, so they feel drier than ever.

Chapped lips are also a sign of internal dehydration, so drinking plenty of liquids can help keep lips smooth and plump. Water or fruit juice is best—coffee, tea and alcohol are not reasonable substitutes.

Sweeten Your Breath Naturally

Ever want to cleanse your palate with some good-breath insurance before an important interview or a big date? Breath mints and mouthwash probably won't help much. Many breath mints contain sugar, on which odor-causing bacteria can feed and multiply.

Brushing your tongue can help to sweeten breath longer and more effectively than mouthwashes. One study showed that while tooth-brushing reduces bacteria-caused mouth odor by up to 38 percent, brushing the teeth *and* tongue reduces odor by up to 76 percent.

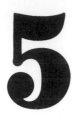

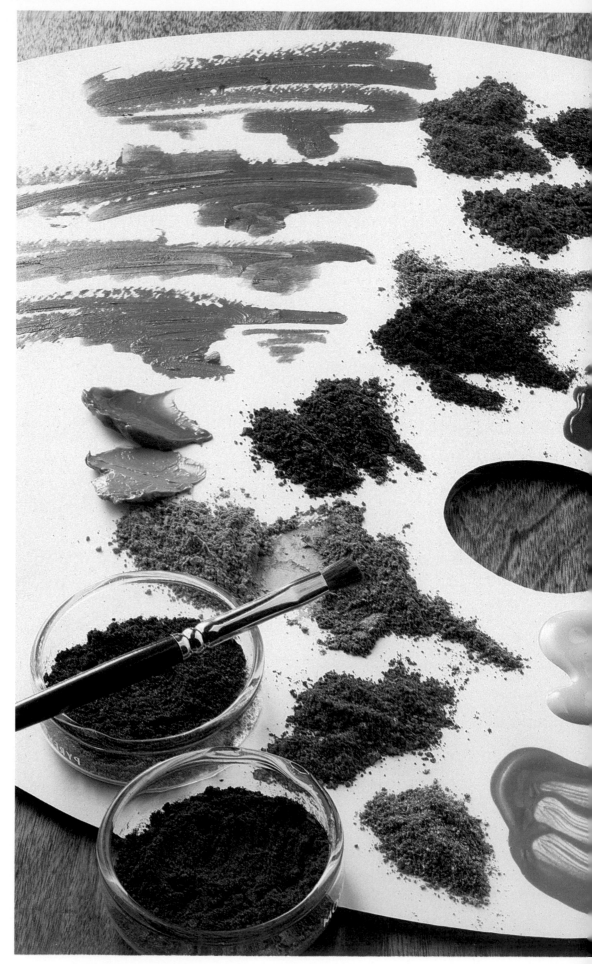

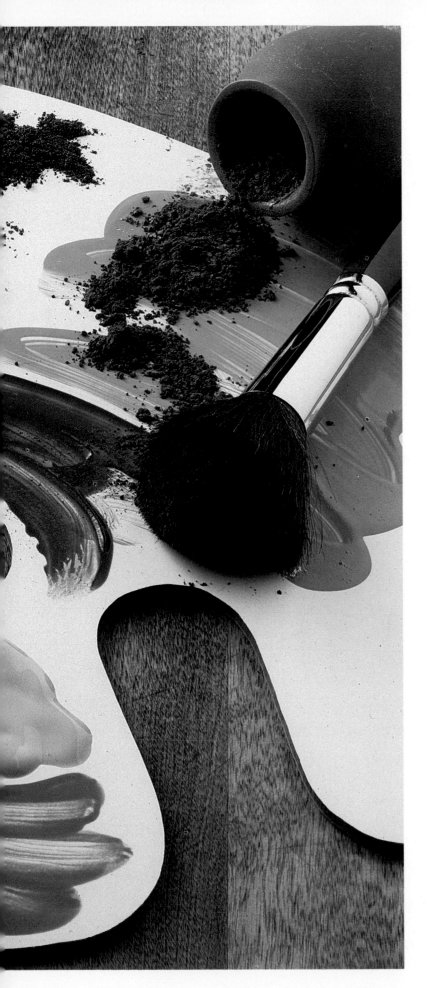

The Art of Makeup

Bring out your beauty with brushes, pencils and a palette of pigments.

Some historians speculate that Richard Nixon would have fared better in a key 1960 presidential campaign debate—and in the subsequent election—if he'd worn makeup on television. When the director/producer of the televised debate offered both Nixon and Senator John Kennedy the services of a staff makeup artist, Senator Kennedy said no, thanks, he had a tan and didn't need any makeup. Nixon heard Kennedy say no, so he refused, too.

In view of his opponent's good looks and charm, Nixon could have benefited greatly from makeup artistry. Ever since that election, political analysts have become aware of the key importance of public image in the literal, visual sense.

Cultivating a public image is important outside the realm of politics, too. Looking one's best can help make anyone a winner. Using makeup artfully is an effective way to enhance your natural features—to "make up" for nature's inequities. And makeup can help improve your self-image as well.

A woman can gain certain psychological benefits from the use of facial makeup, explains Jean Ann Graham, Ph.D., from the department of dermatology at the University of Pennsylvania. She also points out that a woman seems more confident, more organized and more feminine looking, and that wearing makeup helps a woman to feel more sociable, healthier looking, more positive about her self-image and more positive about life.

Like painting and sculpture, makeup artistry depends on the basic principles of proportion, balance, composition and color. For example, there's more to choosing makeup than matching your wardrobe: You should be aware that dark colors can minimize an area and make it appear to recede, while light colors make an area stand out more prominently. Once you understand these and other principles, you can use color and shading to create effects that enhance your best features and play down others.

Double-Duty Makeup

Ordinary foundation makeup and opaque lipstick offer your skin only partial protection against the sun's rays. Because sun damage can cause premature wrinkles, age spots and cancer, every bit of protection helps. So manufacturers now offer foundations and lipstick with built-in sunscreen ingredients such as padimate-O and homosalate to protect you even further. (Sun-blocking lipsticks are just as important as protective foundations, since your lips are as susceptible to sun-induced drying and damage as your skin is.) Makeups rated SPF 15 or higher act as true sun-blocks, multiplying by 15 the time you can spend in the sun without injury.

Foundations

Clinique Continuous Coverage (SPF 19)
Prescriptives Advanced Sun Protection (SPF 19)
Elizabeth Arden Ultra Protection Factor 15 Suncare Sun-Blocking Cream (SPF 15)
Chanel Creme Makeup (SPF 8)
Charles of the Ritz Perfect Protection Makeup (SPF 8)

Lipsticks

Prescriptives Nude Lip Gloss (SPF 12)
Clinique Lip Block (SPF 11)
Max Factor Active Protection Conditioning Lip Gloss (SPF 11)
Estée Lauder Automatic Shine Lipstick (SPF 10)

START WITH A GOOD FOUNDATION

Foundation makeup is flesh-toned cream or lotion that does precisely what its name suggests—it serves as a base for the rest of your makeup. But that's not all it does. Foundation makeup evens out skin tone and texture, hides tiny lines and lends a satiny, dewy or matte finish to skin. Foundation makeup can also enhance your skin below the surface. Products that contain blotting ingredients such as kaolin (a clay powder) or talc soak up excess oil and control shine all day. Foundation creams made with vegetable oil or other emollients seal in moisture for people with dry skin. As an added bonus, foundation makeup shields your face from the damaging effects of sun, wind and pollution.

And you don't have to look like you're wearing a Japanese Kabuki mask to reap all those benefits. The trick is judicious application of a product that's the correct color, weight (or coverage) and finish.

Color. Your skin tone is determined by the combined presence of melanin (brown pigment), carotene (yellow pigment) and the hemoglobin in your blood (red pigment). Dark skin is dominated by brown pigment, sallow skin by yellow pigment, ruddy skin by red pigment. Beige skin is a neutral blend of all three.

Choose a foundation that matches your skin tone as closely as possible, unless you're trying to compensate for an exceptionally ruddy or sallow complexion. If your face usually looks a bit too flushed, a peachy foundation can temper the color. A slightly pinkish foundation adds warmth to a very sallow skin tone. Black skin requires foundation keyed to its undertones: Yellow undertones call for golden shades of foundation, orange undertones need coppery shades and red undertones are enhanced by rose shades.

Coverage. Most people look best in lightweight, lightly tinted foundation. *Sheer foundation* is transparent, revealing as much as possible of your skin's natural tones. *Medium-weight foundation* masks minor imperfections while still allowing your skin to show through. *Full-coverage foundation* conceals most flaws but should be used on trouble spots only, to conceal birthmarks, scars or other variations in pigment. You should coordinate it with a lighter-weight foundation in the same shade for the rest of your face, otherwise it can tend to look artificial. (Cover sticks and concealing creams, blended into your foundation, are especially useful for hiding dark circles.)

Finish. Creams and lotions contain oil and water. The oil helps your foundation spread well. The water evaporates soon after it's applied, leaving a finish that may look dry and nearly invisible or rather moist, depending on how the foundation is formulated. *Matte foundation* usually contains a higher proportion of blotting powder and gives your skin a completely shine-free finish. *Semi-matte foundation* creates a satiny sheen, and *moist foundation* gives a dewy look.

Oiliness. If you have oily or acne-prone skin, the last thing you need is an oily foundation to clog your pores. Look for a foundation with little or no oil. Dry or normal skin does well with a regular oil-based foundation. People with partly oily, partly dry skin (usually referred to as combination skin by skin care professionals) should look for "skin-balancing" foundation makeup.

Reevaluate your foundation makeup from season to season. You may need a lighter-weight, water-based foundation in hot, humid weather and a heavier, moister product in cold, dry weather.

To apply foundation:

- Remove every trace of old makeup or dirt first.
- Dot foundation on your forehead, cheeks, nose and chin and smooth over your entire face—including your eyelids—with a damp cosmetic sponge. (A dry sponge will absorb too much makeup.)
- Blend, blend, blend! You shouldn't be able to tell where your foundation makeup ends and your bare skin begins—and neither should anyone else. Pay special attention to the boundaries at your hairline, earlobes and jaw.

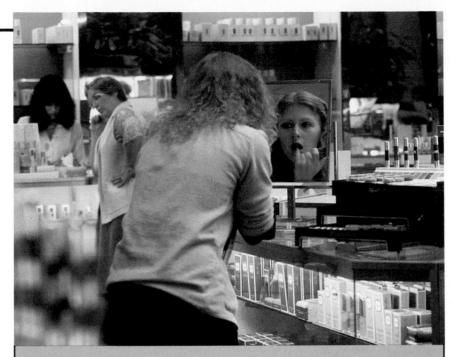

Choosing Colors with Confidence

Testing makeup from display samplers may ensure a perfect color choice but not perfect health— infection-causing bacteria may lurk in those public products. Here's how to choose the right makeup without applying samples directly to your skin.

Foundation. Match the foundation to the skin on the inside of your wrist. Examine the colors in natural light if possible.

Blush. Pinch your cheeks and match the color raised by the blood rushing to the surface of your skin. Fair, ivory or pink-toned complexions generally look best in pinks, roses and heathers. Olive or yellow-toned skins look good in peaches, bronzes and cinnamon. Almost anyone can wear shades of plum since they work well with both warm and cool undertones.

Eye Shadow. Buy an inexpensive multicolor collection and experiment to find out what looks best on you and works well with your wardrobe.

Eyeliner Pencils. Write on the heel of your hand with the sample pencil to get an idea of how the color will look on your lids.

Mascara. This is the one eye makeup that's virtually impossible to try before you buy. But most people can wear either black, brown/black or dark brown, so there's little risk of error if you stick to these basics.

Lip Color. Testing lip color on the heel of your hand doesn't work. Apply it to your lips after first removing a thin layer from the sample tube with a tissue.

FACTS ABOUT BLUSH

Blush is cream, powder or gel formulated to simulate the natural glow your cheeks develop after you exercise or exert yourself, when rich, oxygenated blood swells the otherwise inconspicuous capillaries beneath the skin's surface.

Some women shy away from wearing blush, worried that cheek color will make them look clownish. Delicately applied, though, blush can add interest and dimension to your face, highlighting your individual bone structure and enhancing your skin tone. In fact, the more carefully you choose and apply blush, the more natural the effect. As with foundation, the product you choose depends largely on your skin type and the effect you want to create.

Cream blush contains more oily emollients than do powders or gels and wears well on dry or normal skin, giving a moist, dewy glow. Smooth on cream blush with your fingertips.

Powder blush works fine on all skin types but is most suited to oily skin, because it contains fair amounts of kaolin or other blotting substances. You can apply powder blush with a brush, sponge or puff, but a brush gives you the most control and the softest look of the three.

If you have acne-prone skin, avoid cream or powder blush that contains acetylated lanolin or isopropyl myristate. Both tend to foster blemishes in susceptible people.

Gel blush, applied over foundation or moisturizing lotion, stains

Indispensable Makeup Tools

You'll never have to worry about streaky, blotchy or clumpy-looking makeup if you apply it with the proper tools. Here's everything you'll need for a finished look. *Sharpener with one small hole, one large:* allows fine, precise pencil lines. *Large, fluffy brush:* dusts powder evenly. *Small, slanted, flat brush:* fits eye contour to blend shadow. *Fan-shaped brush:* gives a soft-focus blush. *Lip brush:* gives goofproof definition. *Slant-tipped tweezers:* allow easy brow plucking. *Lash separator/brow brush:* tames brows, declumps mascara. *Latex sponges:* moisten a wedge for even spreading. *Cotton balls and swabs:* buff or whisk away goofs. *Eyelash curler:* makes eyes look wider.

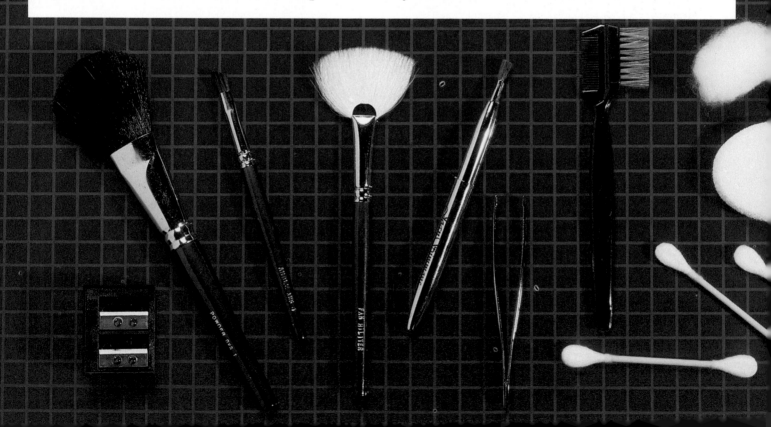

the skin temporarily to create a glossy, transparent glow. Many bronzers, used to simulate a sun-drenched look, come in gel form. Squeeze a small amount onto your fingertips and blend quickly, adding more color if needed. You may have to practice to get a natural effect—most gels contain alcohol, so they evaporate quickly. Consequently, the pigment will stain your skin and look blotchy unless you use plenty of moisturizer and quickly blend a small amount at a time. The alcohol in gels can be drying, so if you have dry skin, you'd be better off using a cream blush.

To determine where you should apply a blush, smile. Then apply blush to the top of the rounded arc of your cheek. Blend well: You should never be able to discern a definite edge to blush color. Above all, use blush sparingly. Better too little than too much.

You can use blush to create flattering contours if you keep in mind two simple principles: Lighter, frosted shades will make your cheekbones appear to come forward; darker, matte shades will make them appear to recede. If you feel that your cheeks look too full and you'd like to bring out hidden cheekbones, you can slim your face and create the illusion of a slight hollow in the center of your cheeks by applying a darker, matte shade of blush below the cheekbone and a slightly lighter, faintly frosted shade to the cheekbone itself, then blending them well. You shouldn't be able to tell where one color begins and the other ends.

Whether you go to the basic blush application or special effects, always check blush color again after you've applied eye and lip colors to be sure all elements look well-balanced.

POWDER: THE OLDEST FORM OF MAKEUP

You can wear powder with or without foundation makeup underneath. Powder helps to blot oil and control shine for people with oily skin, and it can give a soft, smooth, velvety matte finish to any skin tone.

Translucent loose powder is sheer enough to be worn over any foundation and blush—or alone, to allow your skin's natural tones to show through. If you want to use *tinted loose powder,* choose a color one shade lighter than your foundation makeup to compensate for the tendency of tinted powder to darken slightly as it absorbs skin oil. *Frosted powder* sparkles, adding a subtle iridescent glow to your skin on dressy occasions.

To apply loose powder, dip a big, soft, fluffy brush in the powder well, shake off the excess and dust your face with light, even strokes. Whisk away any excess with a fluffy cotton ball.

Pressed powder (applied with a puff) is more heavily textured and more difficult to dust on lightly than loose powder. Pressed powder is

(continued on page 74)

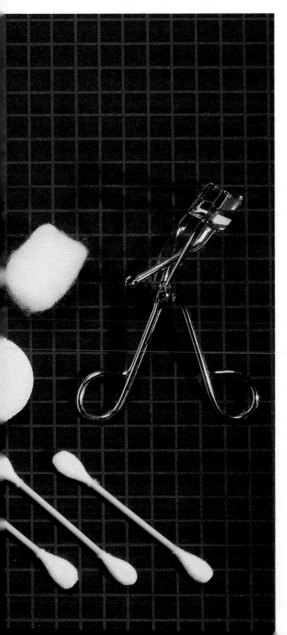

Many lighted makeup mirrors have multiple settings that simulate fluorescent, outdoor and incandescent (bulb) light to help you choose and apply just the right amount and shades of makeup for office, outdoor or home lighting. For example, fluorescent light can give a greenish cast to makeup applied under incandescent lighting. To compensate, use a foundation with a pink tint.

Your Changing Makeup Needs

Chances are, you aren't wearing the same style clothing you wore 10 or 20 years ago. Your makeup, too, should change with your wardrobe, not only to stay in style but to take into account subtle changes your face undergoes as your skin matures.

For example, during the teens and early twenties—considered the acne-prone years—women need to choose the cosmetics least likely to provoke blemishes, according to Glenn Roberts, creative beauty director for Elizabeth Arden, Inc. Women between 20 and 40 have the most freedom of all—their skin is at its peak, and they can wear as little or as much makeup as they like.

But you can still look as fashionable at 40 or 50 as you did at 20. You simply need to compensate for fine lines that appear, especially around the eyes—lines that didn't exist when you were 20.

Roberts emphasizes that women past 45 or 50 need to pay special attention to their makeup. Two pitfalls to avoid: Failing to update makeup to keep in style or trying too hard to hide wrinkles and therefore overdoing makeup.

Colorful, high-fashion makeup may look sensational on a woman in her twenties or thirties but too sophisticated on a 16-year-old and too artificial on a woman in her sixties. By striking a reasonable balance, you can wear makeup to your advantage at any age.

15+ Wear sheer, water-based, oil-free foundation. Use pale eye shadows and one coat of mascara. Don't overpluck brows. Use powder blush for oily skin; otherwise gel blush for a natural glow. Wear translucent lipstick or tinted lip gloss.

20+ Key foundation to skin type; apply lightly. Gear eye shadow to eye color, skin tone, mood. Change to black mascara. Wear conservative powder blush for business, more color for social occasions. Steer clear of garish lip color during the day or for business wear.

30+

Apply foundation a bit more heavily. If wrinkles begin to appear, avoid metallic or frosted eye shadows, which highlight lines. Use more muted shades of blush; keep color away from any facial lines. Use lip liner to prevent lip color from bleeding into dry lines around mouth.

40+

Choose oil-based foundation for dry skin. Apply base lightly over wrinkles, to avoid accentuating lines. Use concealer cream over dark circles, pigmentations. Avoid brash, frosted or metallic shades of eye shadow if lids are puffy. Soften cheek color. Prevent lip color from feathering by using lip base; outline with pencil.

50+

Avoid matte foundation. Avoid iridescent eye shadow or makeup, which emphasizes roughness, crepeyness, lines. Play down puffy lids with gray or smoky shadow, not light shades (which accentuate brow) or reddish tints (which emphasize any redness around eyes). Avoid dark blue-red lipsticks, which are too harsh. Use fresh peach, soft red, warm pink or beigy-rose lip color.

A Makeup Technique for Contact Lens Wearers

Even though having a delicate object in your eye calls for special care in applying makeup, you don't have to give up the finish or the drama of shadows, liners and mascara when you wear contacts. In fact, wear your lenses while you apply your makeup, so you can see what you're doing. (If for some reason you find it difficult to apply makeup while wearing your lenses—and your eyesight is very bad—you might want to invest in magnifying makeup glasses that flip down to correct vision in one eye at a time as you make up your eyes.)

Apply eye shadow with a sponge-tipped applicator rather than a pencil, to put as little pressure as possible on the lens beneath your lid. Also, blot the applicator with a tissue after dabbing it with powder and before applying color to your lids, to remove excess powder that could flake into your eye. Powder trapped underneath the lens could irritate your eye.

Liquid eyeliners are easier to apply than pencil liners, for basically the same reasons. For a soft, subtle, smudged look, gently run a cotton swab along the lid before the liner dries completely.

Use flakeproof and smudgeproof mascara that says on the label it's approved for lens wearers. Avoid mascaras that are supposed to thicken and lengthen lashes considerably—they tend to contain tiny lash-building fibers that can flake into your eyes and lodge underneath your lenses, possibly causing an inflammation.

Remove your eye makeup just as carefully as you apply it. If you wear hard or daily wear soft lenses, remove your lenses before removing your makeup. If you wear extended-wear lenses, avoid oily eye makeup removers—they can irritate eyes and stain lenses. For the same reason, you may want to avoid waterproof mascara, which can't be removed without an oily product. Use cotton balls on the eyelid and cotton swabs along the lash line, dabbing them in oil-free remover, then gently swabbing off eye color.

A REFRESHER COURSE IN EYE MAKEUP

Thanks to advances in cosmetic chemistry—and an overall trend toward soft, natural effects—eye makeup is easier to apply than ever. Eye colors are formulated to last longer even if you play sports or simply have little time to spend in the powder room. Here's a brief inventory of eye makeup products and the special effects you can achieve with each.

Eye shadow works best when applied over concealer or shadow base. Powders, creams and pencils range in color and hues from bare beiges and amazing grays to pastels and vivid, glittery brights. Shadow applied to your upper lids can enlarge your eyes and help ordinary eyes to appear more noticeable and expressive. Muted, gauzy shades tend to look prettier and more natural than bright, frosted shades, especially for daytime wear.

Eyeliner pencils resemble eye shadow pencils. Dark lines drawn along lash lines outline and define the eyes.

Liquid eyeliner, applied with a fine brush, achieves a harder line that's more difficult to blend for soft, subtle effects.

Mascara colors, lengthens and thickens lashes. A spiral brush-tipped wand draws mascara out of a self-contained tube that automatically measures and moistens the makeup for you. These automatic mascaras are convenient and easier to use than cake or cream mascaras, which you apply with a stiff-bristled brush. Moisten the brush with water, rub it on the mascara and stroke onto your lashes from root to tips. Some makeup artists feel that cake or cream mascara makes your lashes look fuller and thicker than do automatic types.

Brow pencils and powders in gray, black or brown can recolor, shape and touch up scanty brows.

FIASCO-PROOF EYE MAKEUP

If you follow our instructions carefully and still aren't satisfied with

great for shine-blotting touchups, though, so tuck a compact in your purse to travel with you.

the way your eye makeup looks, don't despair. Most common goofs can be prevented or corrected.

Eye Shadow Streaks or Creases. You blink about 10,000 times a day. Since eye shadow tends to absorb natural oils from your eyelids, it can easily collect in the folds of the upper lid, forming telltale lines or streaks, especially if you have deep-set eyes or puffy lids.

To help the color last longer, try an eye shadow base such as Elizabeth Arden's Eye Fix or one of its competitors. These creams—combinations of talc, beeswax and other ingredients—form an invisible but protective shield between your eye shadow and skin oils, so the two don't mix and color stays put.

Crooked Eyeliner. Not everyone is skilled with an eyeliner brush. Eyeliner pencils are much easier to work with than liquid liner, especially if you buy soft pencils that glide easily over your lids. If you have crinkly lids or an unsteady hand, try this: Instead of attempting to draw one continuous line, apply a series of closely spaced dots along the lash line, then smudge from corner to corner with a sponge-tipped applicator.

Clumpy or Spiked Mascara. Waterproof mascara clumps less easily than water-based mascara because it dries more slowly, allowing you time to separate lashes. Don't rely on the applicator brush, though. Brush lashes first with a lash separator (see "Ten Indispensable Makeup Tools" on page 70). Apply a thin coat of mascara to lashes, then immediately recomb. Apply a second thin coat after the first coat has dried—about 30 seconds.

Flaky, Smudged or Runny Mascara. In winter, your eyes water. In warm weather, you perspire. Every day, facial oils can wick lash color. Before you know it, you've got raccoon eyes. Waterproof mascara—as the name implies—generally resists smudges better than water-based products, although many water-based mascaras now contain hydrolyzed animal protein or water-based or acrylic resins to help mascara

stay put. To minimize running and streaking, omit foundation makeup on the upper and lower eyelids and pat a narrow streak of eye shadow base (such as Eye Fix) just beneath your lower lashes, then apply mascara. If you find your mascara rubs off or streaks, use a cotton swab to mop up before it dries.

EASY ON, EASY OFF

If your lashes seem to be falling out right before your eyes, be sure that you're removing your makeup correctly. Waterproof mascara requires remover solution that contains mineral oil or similar solvents. If you try to remove waterproof mascara with water, you'll tug and pull your lashes. Instead, soak cotton balls or swabs in oily makeup remover and stroke over the entire lid to remove every trace of eye shadow, liner and mascara. (If the fibers in balls or swabs get caught in your eyes, use makeup remover pads or fiber-free cotton swabs especially designed for removing makeup.) Then gently rub the underside of your lashes until the entire area comes clean when stroked with a fresh cotton ball.

Water-based mascara washes off easily with water and cleansing lotion and is gentler to your lashes in general.

Don't climb into bed at night without removing your eye makeup first: Mascara-coated lashes are somewhat brittle, and if you rub your eyes in your sleep, some lashes are apt to break off.

COLOR-BY-NUMBER LIP PROTECTION

Even if you've been wearing lipstick almost daily since you were in your teens, you probably don't realize that you've been protecting your lips and keeping them plump and healthy while you were adorning your mouth with color.

"Lipstick is more than a beauty aid because it protects the lips from the effects of sun, wind and cold, preventing dryness and chapping," says Charles W. Whitmore, M.D., dermatologist and coauthor of

(continued on page 78)

Doing a Quick Clean-Up

The very ingredients that give your makeup day-long staying power make it difficult to clean off your makeup tools. But the same techniques that remove your makeup can clean those, too.

Use a cotton swab dipped in eye makeup remover or cleansing cream to scrub dried mascara from the rubber pad and frame of your eyelash curler or clean the blade of your eye pencil sharpener. (Be sure to wipe all the cleanser off.) Your makeup brushes are best cleaned by swishing them in warm, soapy water. Rinse them thoroughly. Shake out, reshape the bristles, and let them air-dry in an upright position.

Tips for Perfect Eye Makeup

Subtle touches of eye shadow, liner and mascara following the natural shadows and contours of your eyes can work together to turn your eyes into your most expressive features. Strong colors applied for dramatic effects are best reserved for festive evenings; daytime or outdoor activities call for a light touch and more neutral shades.

Concealer

Begin with concealer to erase undereye circles. Dot and blend it just under the lower lid. Over-lightening accentuates any wrinkles or puffiness and gives you pale, raccoonlike patches under your eyes, so use concealer that's just a shade or two lighter than your natural skin tone. Try yellow-toned concealer to counter bluish circles. Concealer on your lids can also act as a base so your shadow will go on smoothly and adhere longer. Use concealer sparingly; it can cake if applied too heavily.

Shadow

Several thin layers of eye color, blended well, simulate your eyes' natural shadows and contours better than one thick application. Smooth sheer color on the center of each lid with a sponge applicator or soft pencil, then brush up and out toward your brow and in toward your nose with an eye shadow brush. Apply a deep (more intense) shade of color to the crease of your lid and a lighter shade of the same color on the brow bone as a highlighter.

Shaping the Perfect Brow

To shape and refine brows, tweeze one hair at a time. Pluck between the brows (over the bridge of nose) and just beneath them, following each brow's natural arch.

If your brows are skimpy, draw short, feathery lines, in the direction of hair growth (root to tip). Use a sharp brow pencil or powdered eye shadow one shade lighter than your natural brow color. Lightly smudge the lines into your brows with a brow brush.

Ideally, your brows should align over your eyes as shown.

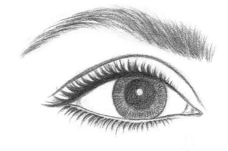

Liner

To define your eyes, outline the top and bottom of the lids close to the lashes. (If you have trouble drawing a straight line, apply closely spaced dots of eyeliner along the base of your lashes.) Line only the outer two-thirds of your upper lids if you have small or deep-set eyes. Smudge the dots or pencil line lightly, from the inner corners outward, for a soft, gradual transition into the eyes' shadows.

Mascara

Stroke each lash separately, from root to tip, holding the wand almost perpendicular to your lids. Allow it to dry between coats.

Understanding Your Skin and Hair. "Lipstick may also protect against cancer of the lip," he adds.

That's because opaque lipsticks shield your lips from the damaging rays of the sun. Glossy, moisturized lip colors prevent windburn, chapping and peeling as well—a boon to athletes and spectators alike.

Choosing and using lipstick was simple back in the 1940s—practically everyone wore some shade of red. Nowadays lip color is more varied, and it's available in pencils and pots as well as tubes. With so many options, even a long-time wearer of lipstick occasionally needs to reevaluate her materials and methods.

To choose the shades that look best on you, keep the following factors in mind.

- Ivory-skinned people look best in peach, salmon or rose lip colors.
- Tawny complexions are complimented by coral, copper or fuschia.
- Olive-toned skin usually calls for shades of brick, nut brown or red.
- Ruddy skin is most flattered by shades of burgundy, sienna (burnt orange) or bronze-toned lip color.
- Black skin is enhanced by plum, mahogany, raisin or red lip colors.

Boost Your Lipstick's Staying Power

Does your lipstick disappear within half an hour after you apply it? Are you too busy for frequent touchups?

If so, look for lipsticks marketed as long wearing. They contain stains that adhere better and longer without irritating the lips the way color dyes used years ago did. The kissproof lipsticks fashionable in the 1950s were durable, but tended to be drying. New dyes give stronger color with less chance of dehydrating or irritating the lips.

Even long-lasting lipsticks can fade too soon, however. Here are some ways to reinforce the staying power of any lipstick.

- Apply foundation makeup underneath lip color, then powder your lips to help the stain adhere and maintain its true shade longer.
- Outline lips in lip pencil the same shade as your lipstick or slightly darker, to hold color within your lip line.
- Apply one coat of lipstick, then blot with a clean tissue. Dust lightly with translucent powder and top with more lipstick to help set color further.
- Smooth on thin top coat of clear lip gloss or plain petroleum jelly.
- Try to avoid pursing or biting your lips, habits which eat away color. And drink beverages through a straw, if convenient.

While you should coordinate your lip color with your clothing, avoid the temptation to match your lipstick to the blouse, sweater or dress you plan to wear. Perfectly matched colors can look artificial and your lipstick will tend to stand out too much. Similarly, your lipstick should harmonize with your cheek color. Peaches, rusts and oranges go together, pinks and plums are related, and red can be worn with shades from either group depending on the tone; deep bluish reds belong to the pink family and coral-reds go with the orange family.

PICTURE-PERFECT LIPS, EVERY TIME

Before applying lip color, prime your lips with a light coat of foundation, then dust with powder. That provides a base to which lip color can adhere so it will last without smudging. Or you can try one of the lip color fixatives on the market, designed to moisturize your lips and prevent the color from "bleeding" into vertical lines.

For precision and accuracy, outline your lips with a lip pencil. The points on hard pencils, made from carnauba wax, paraffin and other stiff wax, hold their shape better than those on soft pencils (or tubes) and prevent lipstick from smearing. Choose a lip pencil that either matches your natural lip color or one that's a shade darker than the lip color you plan to wear.

To outline your lips, relax and smile slightly, with lips closed. Hold the lip pencil as you would a regular writing tool and steady your hand by resting your little finger on your chin. Trace the outer borders, working from the center outward on your upper lip and from the corners inward on your lower lip.

You can use a lip pencil to slightly alter the shape of your mouth or to camouflage minor irregularities (see "Lip Trickery").

Next, use a lip brush to apply your lipstick. Blend the color into the penciled outline so the border looks like a faint shadow, not a hard, distinct line. Don't roll your upper and lower lips together to set the

Lip Trickery

If you're not perfectly satisfied with the shape of your mouth, you can reshape your lips with lipstick. (Don't try to radically reshape your mouth, though, or you'll look silly.)

To make narrow lips appear fuller: Outline your mouth, then fill in with light to medium lip color—mocha, peach or dusty rose, for example. To heighten the effect, use frosted and glossy lip colors and apply a slightly lighter shade to the center of the lower lip. They reflect light, adding additional fullness.

To deemphasize very full lips: Extend your foundation makeup over your lips. Draw an outline of both lips just inside their margins. Fill in with a single shade.

color, no matter what your mother may have told you. You'll only smear a perfect paint job.

Using a lip pencil and brush takes more time than simply using a lipstick tube, but together they enable you to apply lipstick more evenly and accurately, especially after the tapered end of the lipstick tube wears down. A lip brush also extends the useful life of lipstick because you can reach that last quarter inch or so of the stick. A lip brush is also indispensable for blending two shades of lipstick into a new, flattering shade, multiplying your options from just two or three basic tubes of color. They make wearing lipstick creative, fun *and* economical.

If you know you're allergic to the lanolin in moisturizing lotions or foundation makeup, be aware that lanolin in lipstick may leave your lips dry and cracked. Switching to a lanolin-free brand of lip color should solve this problem.

(continued on page 84)

Contouring with a Light Touch

You can bring out your best features (or play down your flaws) by applying the same principles that a painter uses to make the picture on a flat canvas appear three-dimensional. Light colors make surfaces appear larger or closer to the viewer; dark colors make surfaces appear smaller or more distant. That means pale or glossy makeup, which reflects light, can bring out your best features. And dark, matte makeup will minimize large features or provide contrast that will emphasize your highlights. You can work this magic with foundations or blushers a shade or two lighter or darker than your natural skin tone.

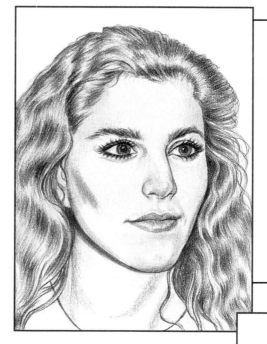

Show Off Your Cheekbones

Emphasizing your cheekbones also draws attention to your eyes. Apply highlights over your cheekbones, no closer than a finger's width from your eyes and nose and no lower than your nostrils. Hollow your cheeks with shading just beneath the cheekbone. Blend carefully.

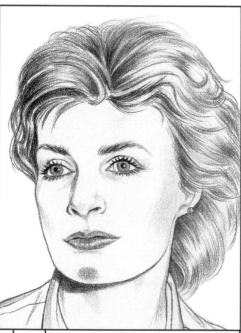

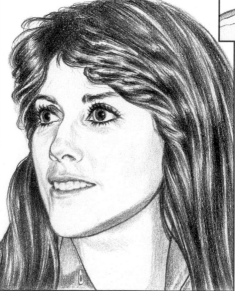

Downplay Your Jaw

To soften a strong jawline, apply a contour shadow cream or deeper-toned blush along and just beneath your jawbone. Blend carefully with sponge or brush.

Make More of Your Chin

To create the illusion of a fuller chin, apply a spot of light foundation, concealer cream or highlighting cream to the center of a receding chin.

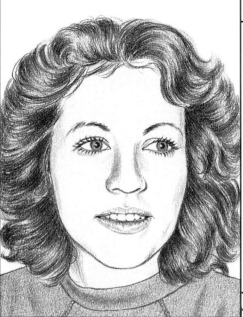

Slim Your Nose

Using a small brush, apply a narrow stripe of pale foundation, highlighting cream or powder from bridge of nose to tip. Then shadow the sides of your nose with makeup a shade darker than your foundation. Blend carefully. (Reverse the technique to widen a narrow nose.) As with most contouring techniques, this takes practice to look convincing.

Contour Tips

- Use contour shading and highlights sparingly. Better too little than too much.
- Blend color well to soften lines of demarcation and give a subtle, natural look to contours.
- To balance the color on your cheekbones with the makeup on the rest of your face, blend a touch of blush at the center of your forehead and chin, using circular motions.
- Check the color again after you've applied your eye and lip color to be sure you've applied proportionate amounts of color to your eyes, cheeks and lips so that no one feature dominates your face.

Soften Your Forehead

Place dots of dark foundation or contour cream from temple to temple along your hairline. Blend into foundation. Dust with translucent powder to prevent shine.

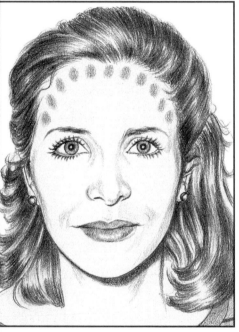

Slim a Wide Face

Look in a mirror and superimpose an imaginary oval over your face. Then smooth a dark contouring shade along that part of your face that falls outside the sides of the oval. Blend well.

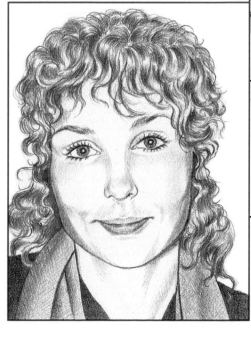

Step by Step to a More Beautiful Face

New York makeup artist Joe Oliver reached into his bag of tricks to show you how all aspects of makeup—color, contouring and highlighting—work together to make the most of anyone's features. Joe chose colors geared specifically for the model's pink skin undertones and pale complexion. And he artfully applied color to widen Allison's close-set eyes and soften her squarish face. You can use the same basic principles, explained with each step, when applying your own makeup.

"There's a lot going on here, but it all works together to create a livelier, prettier look. All you need is a little practice," says Joe.

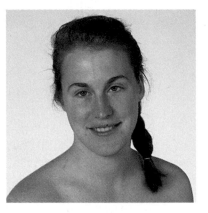

To begin, Joe cleansed and moisturized Allison's face. Applying a moisturizer allows you to use a water-based foundation makeup, which is less apt to clog pores and cause blemishes than an oil-based foundation.

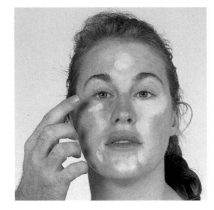

Joe patted off-white highlighting cream on Allison's midforehead, under her eyes, over the creases along her nose and mouth and on her chin to hide blemishes and undereye circles and to create highlights from which to work further. He thoroughly blended the cream into her skin, working toward her nose.

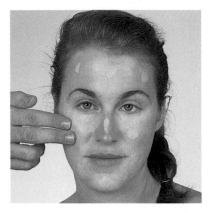

Next, Joe dotted on a light beige foundation with a hint of pink to further even out Allison's skin tones and perk up her pale complexion. Using a damp sponge, always blend foundation well, especially at your jawline and neck.

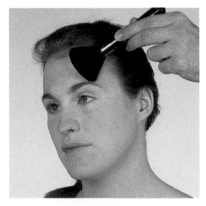

Next he dusted on loose translucent powder with a large powder brush to set makeup, blot oil and give skin a matte (nonshiny) finish. Joe chose a light pink-beige for Allison to complement her pink undertones.

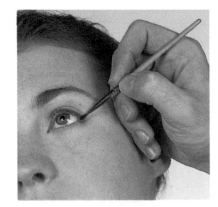

The artist used a small, fine-tipped brush to apply black powder eyeliner to Allison's lids. Here, he blends liner with a medium brush.

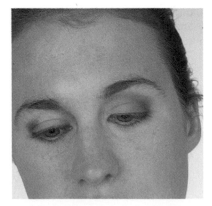

To make Allison's eyes appear larger and farther apart, Joe applied raisin-colored shadow above the crease of each eye, no closer to her nose than the point above each pupil and stopping short of her brow bones. To blend the shadow, he lightly dusted a sheer layer of light pink powder across the entire eyelid.

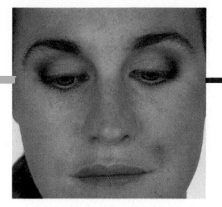

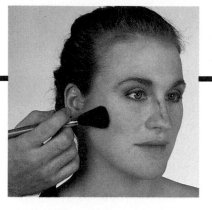

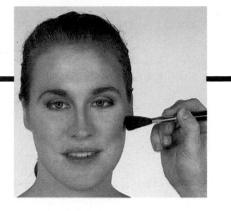

To further enlarge and widen Allison's eyes, Joe then superimposed a slight smudge of sheer black shadow toward the outer corner of each eye. To enlarge her eyes still further, he swept a slight hint of gold from the inner to the outer edge of the eyelid, up to the brow bone.

To sharpen Allison's nose and emphasize her bone structure, Joe applied a thin streak of dark contour cream along each side of her nose and light pink contour cream to her cheeks. Both were blended well.

To apply blush, Joe dusted powder blush on the ball of Allison's cheek—the mound formed when you say "sing"—and blended the color using circular strokes. Joe also applied blush to the outer edges of Allison's forehead to help her squarish face appear oval.

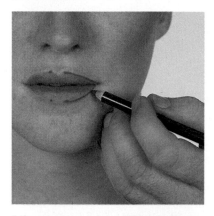

Joe filled in Allison's lip color with a shade of pink that flattered her pink-toned skin. To add fullness to her lower lip, he brushed on clear lip gloss.

Like many people's, Allison's lips aren't perfectly symmetrical. To apply lipstick evenly, Joe recommends applying four dots of color with a lip pencil, as shown here, and then outlining the lips by connecting the dots and the corners of the lips.

A touch of black mascara, plus a 20-minute set with electric curlers and a comb-out was all that remained to complete Allison's makeover.

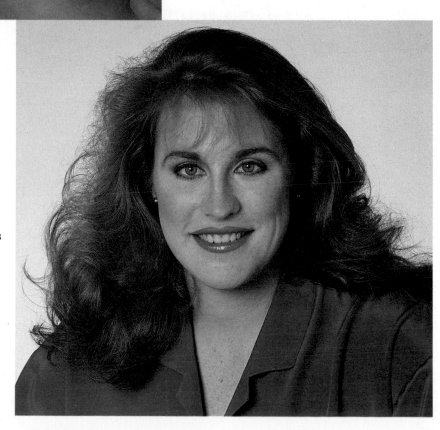

MAKEUP: SAFER THAN EVER

In the late 18th century, women coated their skin with a poisonous lead compound known as ceruse to impart the pale complexions that were fashionable then. Because skin absorbs anything applied to it, the cosmetic gave a whole new meaning to the phrase *femme fatale*.

Today, thanks to modern cosmetic chemistry, women no longer have to sacrifice their health for beauty's sake.

Many people believe that cosmetics undergo rigorous tests for safety by the U.S. Food and Drug Administration before they're marketed. In fact, just the opposite is true: The FDA investigates consumer complaints and develops regulations (such as requiring manufacturers to list ingredients), but the agency leaves the responsibility for safety to cosmetic manufacturers—primarily because only 1 percent of the FDA budget is allotted to cosmetics.

When it comes to obvious, immediate reactions such as irritation or allergies, self-regulation seems to work fairly well. Companies routinely test each and every ingredient for its ability to irritate skin, first on animals, then on people. As a result, millions of people use dozens of products containing any of 4,000 or so ingredients daily, and of about 500 cosmetic-related complaints received by the FDA in a recent year, only about 4 percent involved facial makeup. This seems remarkable when you consider that your face and eyes are among the most sensitive parts of the body and that cosmetics remain on the skin for hours at a time. Usually the reactions that do occur are so minor—

What's in Your Makeup

Understanding the functions of the ingredients listed on your makeup labels will do more than satisfy idle curiosity—it can help you choose the cosmetics best suited to your skin type or track down the cause of an allergic reaction.

More than 4,000 possible ingredients go into makeups—far too many to enumerate here. Most of these ingredients tend to fall into one of the categories shown in the chart at right. (Categories overlap occasionally, as you'll note on the chart.)

The *base* of a cosmetic is the main ingredient in which other ingredients are mixed. *Emollients* are oils that help retain your skin's moisture and prevent the makeup itself from drying too much once it's on your face. *Emulsifiers* homogenize ingredients that don't ordinarily mix, like oil and water. They prevent the makeup from separating and help it spread well. *Waxes* provide body and texture and help makeup adhere to your skin. *Pigments* supply the shades in your makeup. They are derived from petroleum, minerals or plants. The U.S. Food and Drug Administration considers relatively few pigments safe enough to include in makeup, with the fewest permitted in eye and lip formulations. In addition, makeups contain *fillers* to improve texture and *oil blotters* to reduce your skin's oily shine. Except for eye makeup, most cosmetics contain small amounts of *fragrance*. Virtually all makeup contains *preservatives* to prevent rancidity, deterioration and bacterial contamination.

Makeup	Base (Main Ingredient)	
Foundation	Water or oil	
Blush and powder	Talc, kaolin, water	
Eye shadow	Talc, calcium carbonate	
Eyeliner	Cocoa butter with mineral or vegetable oil; styrenebutadiene latex and water	
Mascara	Water (water-based); petroleum distillates (solvent-based)	
Lipstick	*See* Waxes	

mild burning, stinging or itching—that most people don't even bother to report them to their doctor. They simply switch brands and hope for the best. But why suffer at all? If cosmetics irritate your skin despite the manufacturers' efforts, you can avoid further problems by learning to recognize and avoid the cause.

ALLERGY, IRRITATION OR INFECTION?

Allergic reactions are the most common adverse effects of cosmetics. Redness, swelling and itching may occur 12 to 48 hours after you've applied a product, even if you've used it uneventfully for years. Irritation can also cause burning, itching and stinging as well as welts, red blotches that resemble bruises, blisters or an eczemalike rash.

Don't worry if you can't tell whether you're experiencing an allergy or an irritation—doctors say they can't always tell the difference, either. It's more important to identify the cause of the reaction and know what to do about it than to know what to call it, according to Dr. Albert Kligman, a leading expert on skin problems.

Allergic reactions or irritation from cosmetics are usually triggered by three categories of ingredients: fragrances (including balsam of Peru, musk ambrette, cinnamic aldehyde and hundreds of others); emollients

Emollient (Oil)	Emulsifiers (Binders)	Waxes	Colors
Lanolin, mineral oil, silicone oil, vegetable oils and esters of fatty acids	Glycerol stearate or other stearic compounds, triethanolamine and polyoxyethylene fatty acid esters	Wool wax alcohol, carnauba wax, cetyl alcohol, beeswax or other waxes	Mineral oxides such as zinc oxide and iron oxide; inorganic (carbonless) compounds such as ultramarine blue (for muted shades) and titanium dioxide (for even coverage)
Mineral oil, lanolin, vegetable oils	Zinc stearate	Paraffin, beeswax, carnauba wax	Red, yellow and brown iron oxides, organic (carbon-based) colors such as carmine, D&C Red Nos. 7, 9, 19, 30 (for vivid shades), titanium dioxide
Petrolatum, mineral oil, lanolin	Sorbitan, oleate	Paraffin, beeswax, mineral wax such as ceresin or ozokerite	The pigments used in eye cosmetics are iron oxides (for earth tones), titanium dioxide (for pastels), ultramarine blue, pink and violet (for muted shades), copper, silver and aluminum powders (for metallic shades), carmine (for bright reds), manganese violet, chrome oxide, chrome hydrate, ferric ferrocyanide, bismuth oxychloride, mica, talc
Vegetable oil derivatives	Triethanolamine stearates and polyoxyethylene fatty acid esters	Japan wax with beeswax, carnauba wax, ceresin or ozokerite, fatty alcohols	See Eye shadow
None	Glycerol stearate, triethanolamine (water-based); aluminum stearate or polyethylene (solvent-based)	Beeswax, carnauba wax, ozokerite	See Eye shadow
Isopropyl palmitate and other fatty acid compounds, mineral oil, cetyl alcohol and other fatty alcohols, castor oil, lanolin, hydrogenated vegetable oils	Stearates	Lanolin wax, beeswax, carnauba wax, candelilla wax, rice wax and other natural waxes	Pigments and dyes allowed in lipstick include iron oxides, titanium dioxide, FD&C Blue No. 1, D&C Red Nos. 6, 7, 8, 9, 17, 21 and 36, FD&C Red Nos. 3 and 30, D&C Orange No. 5, FD&C Yellow Nos. 5 and 6

How Safe Is Your Makeup?

Like food, makeup is perishable. But because makeup is not labeled with expiration dates the way, say, dairy products are, it's up to you to store and use makeup carefully to prolong its "shelf life." If you don't, even cosmetics with preservatives can spoil: They can cake, dry out, turn color or—worst of all—become contaminated with infectious bacteria.

And that's especially true of eye makeup—liners, mascaras and shadows. "Using the same applicator day after day reintroduces bacteria from your eye to the product and vice versa," says Gail Bucher, past president of the Society of Cosmetic Chemists and corporate quality analyst for Gillette, a leading manufacturer of cosmetics and other personal care products. "The eyes are very sensitive organs. Eye infections can be extremely severe—possibly causing blindness. So consumers have to be very careful."

To avoid this problem, use disposable eye shadow applicators—cotton swabs—or washable sponge applicators. Also, label shadow, pencils and mascara with the purchase dates. Replace your shadow and pencils every 6 months and your mascara every 3 months. (Keep them longer than that and their preservatives may not be fully effective in fending off bacteria.)

Don't store eye shadow (or contour, pressed or loose powder) in a steamy area such as the bathroom. Powdery products cake easily in excess humidity.

As for lipsticks, foundation and cream blushers, keep them out of the sun and don't expose them to heat or near-freezing temperatures. The chemicals in oil- and water-based products can break down when exposed to bright light or extreme heat or cold.

And a rule for all makeup: When in doubt, throw it out. If you notice a change in the color or smell of a cosmetic, get rid of it.

amount of trial and error. Some ingredients will cause a reaction only when combined with certain other ingredients. Or they will cause stinging or itching around the eyes but not on the cheeks, which are less sensitive. (See "How to Head Off Allergic Reactions to Makeup" for additional tips on avoiding troublesome cosmetics.) Above all, don't continue to use any product that irritates you, thinking you'll get used to it. The problem will only get worse.

Often cosmetic ingredients themselves are innocent of blame. Used carelessly, certain cosmetics can harbor bacteria that lead to infections. For example, small numbers of bacteria such as *Staphylococcus epidermis* and *S. aureus* peaceably inhabit the eye area. When picked up by mascara or other eye makeup products, those bacteria feed on the rich emollients and grow by leaps and bounds. Preservatives such as parabens keep bacteria in check—up to a point. Misusing the product or storing makeup carelessly can cause makeup to deteriorate or become contaminated. (Preservatives can lose their effectiveness after three months or so.) To prevent makeup-induced infections, observe the following precautions.

- Wash your hands before applying cosmetics. Otherwise, you risk introducing dirt and bacteria to your eyes.
- Keep cosmetic containers clean. Wipe off dust and smudges with a damp cloth to avoid contamination.
- Never apply eye makeup when you're riding in a moving vehicle. You risk scratching your cornea, the eyes' protective covering, which could provide a cozy niche for bacteria to enter your eye, possibly causing loss of sight.
- If you have an eye infection or the skin around the eye is inflamed, wait until the problem heals completely before using any eye makeup.
- Never try to smooth out clumpy mascara with saliva. The bacteria from your mouth may flourish in the mascara and contaminate your eyes.

(such as lanolin and butyl stearate); and preservatives (such as methylparabens and sorbic acid).

Nailing down the cause of a cosmetic reaction requires a certain

- Never thin old mascara with water—that dilutes the preservatives. Buy a fresh tube instead.

RISK VS. BEAUTY BENEFIT

While the cosmetic industry has done a commendable job of monitoring makeup safety and preventing injuries, the issue of long-term safety is not quite so simple. For example, triethanolamine (TEA), an emulsifier used in foundation and eye makeup as well as in shampoos, lotions, perfumes and other grooming products, is in itself harmless. But TEA and similar amine compounds react with other ingredients in makeup to form n-nitrosodiethanolomine (NDELA), a compound known as a nitrosamine. Like the nitrosamines formed by nitrites in bacon and other cured meats, nitrosamines in makeup have been shown to cause cancer in laboratory animals. So have D&C Red Nos. 9 and 19, dyes used in lipstick. Of course, no one is positive that all chemicals that cause cancer in animals also cause cancer in people. Health risks are also related to how much of a suspicious ingredient people have to be exposed to—and for how long—before suffering harm.

At this writing, the FDA is seriously considering a ban on the following color additives in cosmetics: FD&C Red No. 3, FD&C Yellows Nos. 5 and 6, D&C Red Nos. 8, 9, 19, 33, 36, 37 and D&C Orange No. 17.

As with therapeutic drugs, the safety of cosmetics comes down to two matters: finding acceptable alternatives to questionable ingredients and balancing benefit against risk. Makeup and other grooming products that do not include TEA or other questionable ingredients are available and are usually found in the health food section of stores and supermarkets. Unfortunately, the selection of colors and products in these lines may be more limited than in the larger, better-known brands.

Many people—consumers and cosmetic researchers alike—feel that the real psychological and emotional benefits of wearing makeup outweigh the suspected but remote and unconfirmed risks of a few questionable ingredients. Keep in mind that few products are absolutely safe. In fact, Congress has abandoned use of the term "safe" in consumer legislation and prefers to describe products as posing "no reasonable risk," to emphasize the need to balance risk against benefit.

Zenona W. Mally, M.D., a clinical assistant professor of dermatology at Georgetown University, sums up the safety issue by saying, "Today's cosmetics are among the safest products available to the public, but they must be used wisely and must be used for their intended purpose. No rules, regulations or precautions by government or industry can protect the person who does not read the label and follow directions and warnings."

How to Head Off Allergic Reactions to Makeup

Makeup is supposed to cover blotches, not create them, yet every so often a product can spring a nasty surprise in the form of an allergic reaction. Even a brand of makeup you've used for years can suddenly cause hives and swelling or make your eyes sting or your nose run. Such outbreaks are unpredictable to some extent, but there are some shopping tips to reduce the likelihood of allergic reactions.

- Look for makeup labeled "hypoallergenic." This label means the product has been scientifically proven to cause fewer allergic reactions than comparable products not specially formulated for people with allergies.
- Steer clear of makeup that contains fragrance, the number one troublemaker for sensitive skin.
- Don't be tempted to buy a whole line of a brand of makeup you've never used before. Ask for a free application or buy a sample size, then wait a few days to see if you experience a delayed reaction.

Natural Meets Synthetic. Best of Both Worlds

Plant and animal products have been used as bases, colors and fragrances in makeup since ancient times. Today, some people believe that products that come from the earth instead of a lab are somehow gentler and more compatible with our skin than synthetics.

But natural products aren't always better than synthetics. For example, most makeup contains water, which fosters bacterial growth. Natural preservatives, such as rosemary oil and grapefruit seed extract, don't prevent contamination nearly as well as synthetic compounds such as parabens.

Moreover, synthetic ingredients also can help natural ingredients perform better. For example, sesame oil and water don't mix, but adding a synthetic emulsifier such as propyl glycol monostearate binds them together into a rich, spreadable foundation makeup base.

The substances shown here are examples of natural ingredients that perform valuable roles in cosmetics, often aided by synthetic compounds.

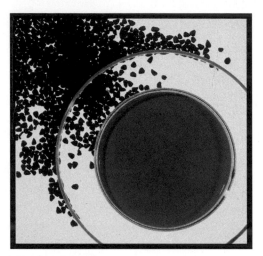

Annatto

A yellow-red dye derived from the seed of a tropical shrub. Used to color some cosmetics.

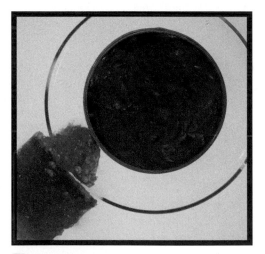

Beeswax

A base for lipstick and foundation makeup.

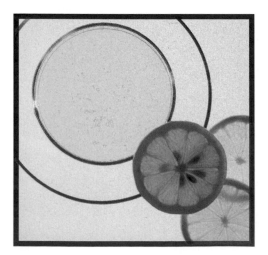

Citric Acid

Derived from lemons or limes. Used as a fragrance or preservative in makeup.

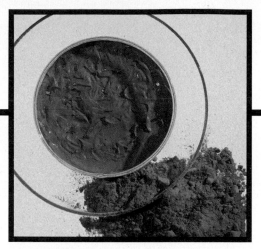

Kaolin

A mineral used in face powder
and eye shadow to absorb oil
and in mascara to thicken lashes.

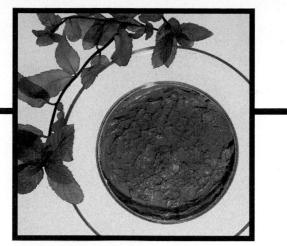

Menthol

An oil synthesized or derived
from peppermint and other mints.
Soothes the skin.

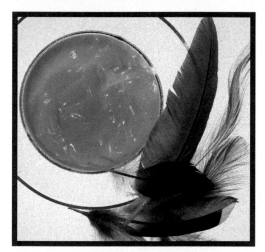

Keratin

A protein derived from horns,
hooves and feathers. Used in
conditioning products.

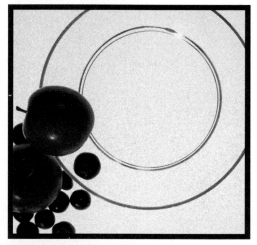

Sorbitol

Derived from berries, cherries,
plums and pears. Attracts moisture and helps skin to feel smooth.

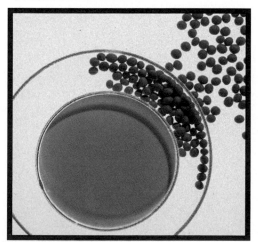

Lecithin

Derived from soybeans. Used in
cosmetics to bind ingredients
together and prevent rancidity.

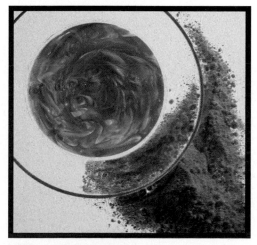

Zinc Oxide

A powdery mineral used to
clean and protect the skin.

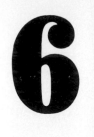

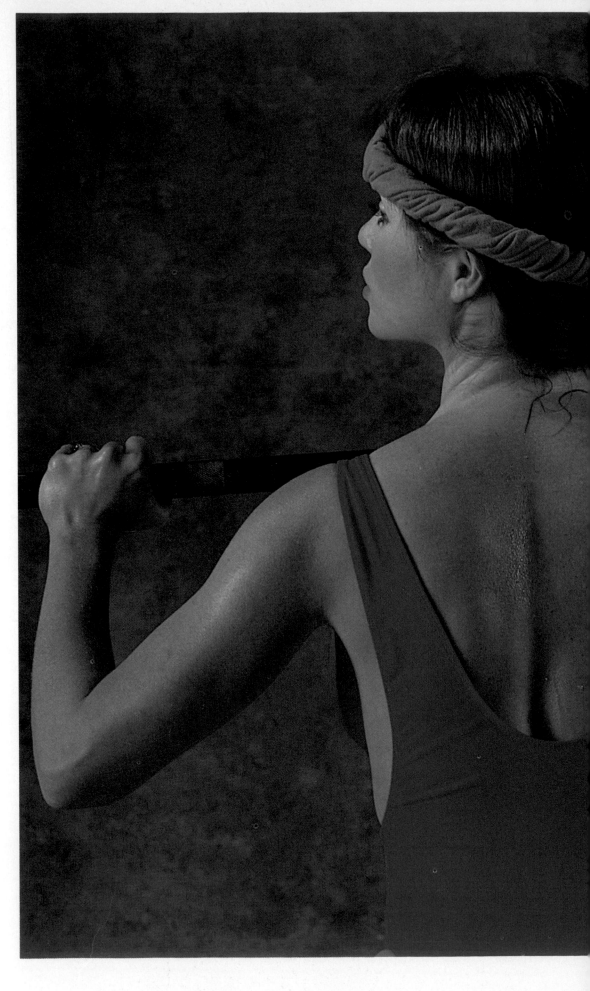

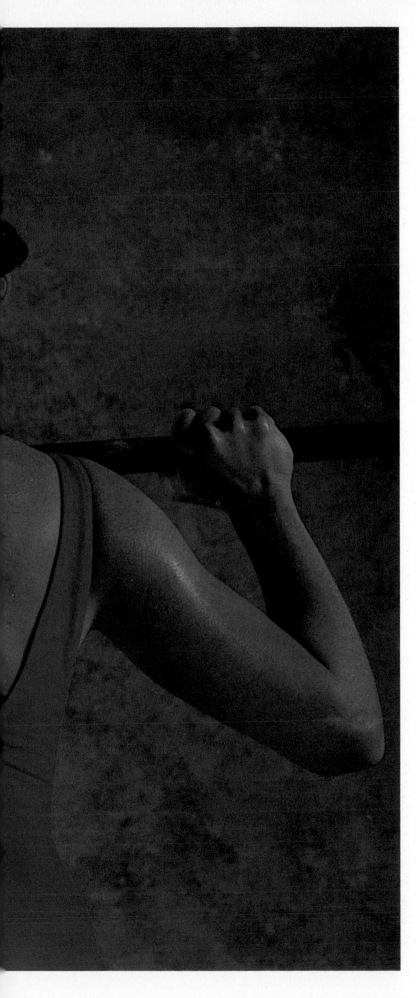

Shaping Up

Exercise propels you toward enhanced health—and better looks—in the same motion.

W hy, oh why do people crowd into those heart-pumping aerobics classes and work up such a sweat? Or pump iron down at the health club? Or jog through the park, rain or shine, when it would be easier to sack out on the sofa?

One answer is health. But another answer—just as compelling—is beauty. Men and women work out to work toward the body beautiful, to achieve better looks by firming up muscles, burning off flab and building up self-confidence. And exercise scientists are nodding in approval as the evidence for the fitness/beauty connection mounts up.

The experts are also saying that it may be far easier to get into shape than you think—because they've been helping to revise the idea of what a good shape is. For years the "ideal weight" charts handed out by doctors and displayed on drugstore scales told people they were too fat for their own good. But now many authorities are saying that such charts give people the wrong impression.

"It's very deceiving to use height and weight tables to figure out what shape you're in," says Grant Gwinup, M.D., professor and acting chairman of the division of endocrinology and metabolism at the University of California at Irvine. "They don't tell you enough. According to a chart, two people can both be at an 'ideal' weight, but one may be all muscle while the other is all flab. How much you weigh doesn't mean as much for your health as the amount of body fat you carry."

In addition, although standard weight charts try to tell you that you should weigh the same throughout your adult life, research shows that if there is such a thing as an ideal weight, it increases as you get older.

Certainly medical professionals recognize that being grossly overweight is a health hazard, but some of them are also saying that striving to meet some arbitrary weight or shape standard can be a frustrating, pointless struggle. It's far more important to be in the best physical shape possible for your build. Being in shape—regardless of your shapeliness—is always attractive. And that's where exercise comes in.

WHAT EXERCISE CAN DO FOR YOU

It has taken more than a decade of research to confirm what fitness buffs already knew: Exercise not only improves your insides but enhances your outsides as well. For those who aspire to the body beautiful, working out has never had more proven advantages.

Chief among the pluses is exercise's power to shift your body's balance of fat and muscle. You already know that physical activity burns fat (and that in itself is a nice thing to note in the mirror), but you should also realize that working out increases muscle mass, too. This burning and building process changes your fat-to-muscle ratio—which in turn can alter how you look in a bathing suit.

You see, a pound of muscle is more densely packed than a pound of fat, so it's smaller. Thus a shift toward increased muscle and decreased fat can mean a slimmed-down appearance. A 135-pound woman, for example, could actually go down a dress size without losing a pound.

And according to recent research, exercise is the *only* way you can accomplish this trick of building muscle while discarding fat. We now know that people who diet without exercise burn a lot of muscle along with the fat—a process that may not be at all kind to your figure.

Muscle and fat don't just sit there and take up space—they use up calories. But muscle mass at rest burns more calories than fat does. Which means that by adding muscle through exercise, you can increase your basal metabolic rate (the speed at which your body burns calories at rest) and thus hurry along the rate at which you shed extra pounds.

Then there's the body shaping that comes from toning, the stretching and strengthening of muscle old or new. Such movement is fundamental in the fitness world, but not everyone realizes just how much toning can do for the human physique.

Ellington Darden, Ph.D., exercise expert and author of *The Nautilus Woman,* points out that stretching and strengthening the right muscles can reduce flabbiness on the buttocks and hips, give greater definition to thighs and calves, make shoulders appear broader or less bony, improve the contours of the midsection, enhance erect and confident posture, even give more poise to sagging breasts. And no doubt hundreds of other fitness experts would concur—and add a list of visual benefits of their own. It's simple common sense that by improving the function of muscles, their form naturally improves.

What's good for muscle is also good for bone. Scientific evidence suggests that exercise can actually increase the size and density of bones, the inner foundation for our outward appearance. Such news becomes increasingly welcome as we

---

Is Thinner Better?

If you lose unsightly extra pounds you'll *look* better. But will you actually be healthier?

The answer seems to be yes. A major report released by the National Institutes of Health in 1985 concluded that:

- People whose weight is 20 percent or more above the "ideal" weights recommended by the Metropolitan Life Insurance Company run a higher risk of heart disease, diabetes and cancer.
- The more you exceed the desirable weight range, the less your chances of living as long as you normally would.
- If you gain extra weight in your 20s, 30s or 40s, your health risks are higher than if you put on those few pounds after age 50.

What do these sets of facts mean? Say you're a medium-framed woman standing 5'6'' in 1-inch heels and you weigh 172 pounds—20 to 30 percent more than the 130 to 144 pounds recommended for your sex and height. Losing weight will probably add healthy years to your life.

Don't worry if you're *under*weight: Being thin is a hazard only if you smoke, if your periods cease before menopause, if you have anorexia nervosa (an eating disorder), or if you involuntarily lose a lot of weight—all associated with specific health risks.

age, for getting older usually means slowly losing bone mass. When this destruction is accelerated—as it is most frequently in older women—it's called osteoporosis. It's what turns women with good carriage into stooped "little old ladies." Exercise, however, seems to counteract such postural damage.

Everett L. Smith, Ph.D., assistant clinical professor of preventive medicine at the University of Wisconsin in Madison, is one of several researchers who has demonstrated the bone-building power of physical activity. In one study he found that people who exercised regularly for three years achieved a 2.3 percent *increase* in bone mineral mass, while a comparable group of people who didn't exercise had a 3.3 percent *decrease* in bone mineral mass.

"The idea is to keep moving," says Dr. Smith. "Even a little bit of exercise is better than none, whether it's aerobic or not. Just 30 minutes a day of walking or dancing will help stabilize the rate of bone loss due to aging."

"Exercise can benefit the skin the same way it benefits the bones and the muscles," says Dr. Albert Kligman, of the Hospital of the University of Pennsylvania. "Without exercise, the bones get brittle and the muscles shrink. Likewise, the skin gets thinner, less elastic and less able to protect against the environment."

The principal evidence of the exercise/skin connection comes from studies of athletes. It's been shown that their skin is thicker and has more collagen (the main source of skin's elasticity) than that of non-athletes. But perhaps even more persuasive is the effect often noticed by exercise's loyal practitioners: a greatly improved complexion.

Exercise is also preventive medicine for the unsightly disorder known as varicose veins, a disease afflicting one in four American women and one in ten American men. "In varicose veins, the veins have lost their elasticity and are stretched out of shape, and the valves are not functioning properly," says Howard C. Baron, M.D., attending vascular surgeon at the Cabrini Medical Center in New York City and author of

Varicose Veins: A Commonsense Guide to Their Management. Sooner or later, he says, blood pools and stagnates in the veins, which further dilates the vessels. The result of all this is the familiar roadmap of gnarled blue ropes.

But, some experts say, exercise can reduce the risk or help prevent the complications of such a condition. Dr. Baron points out that contracting muscles in the calves forces blood in the veins upward, lessening the chance of blood pooling. And other physicians say that an exercise as simple as walking can reduce blood pressure in veins to about a third of the pressure present while standing.

So the prescription is movement. "Walk, run, jump or jog," says Dr. Baron. "Do anything to keep those legs moving."

We often equate being in shape with looking and feeling younger—and with good reason. Your fitness level is better than your birth certificate as an indicator of age. Take the people in this photo, for instance. Can you tell how old they are from the way they look in leotards? Turn the page for the answers.

Question

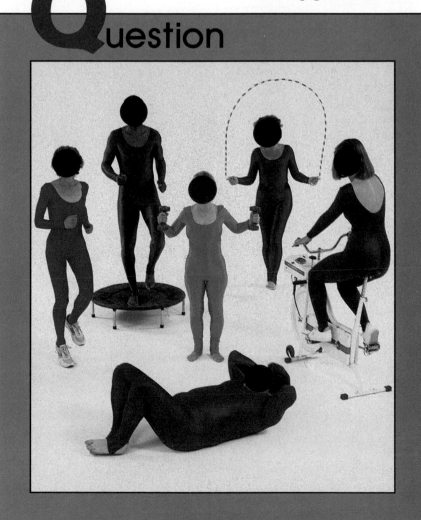

93

Exercise can make you look happy because it makes you feel happy. When you're depressed, anxious or stressed, you don't look as good as you could. Change the way you feel and you change the way you look. Research indicates that exercising releases a hormone called noradrenaline into your system and thus elevates your mood. Noradrenaline causes the body to release another substance which some scientists believe may be responsible for the much talked-about "runner's high." Moving your muscles helps to dispel the tension that builds up in them due to stress.

Some of the evidence for exercise's positive effect on your feelings comes from the University of Wisconsin Medical School in Madison. Doctors there asked ten depressed and socially isolated men to exercise 45 to 60 minutes twice a week for 30 weeks. At the end of the study the men were stronger, showed more stamina and had lower blood pressure and resting heart rates—just the kind of physical changes you'd expect. But the men had also experienced an emotional makeover: They were clearly more hopeful and less anxious, resulting in an improved sense of well-being.

THE RIGHT EXERCISE FOR YOU

The best exercise programs, say the experts, invariably include three kinds of activity: aerobic conditioning that vigorously works your heart and lungs, muscle strengthening, and stretching for flexibility. You need aerobic conditioning to give you stamina, to lessen fatigue, to help you gain all the health benefits that come from improving your heart and lungs. You need strengthening workouts to reduce your risk of lower back pain and injuries to bones and soft tissues. And you need flexibility training to give you freedom of movement.

Unfortunately, no single exercise incorporates all three forms of movement to maximum degrees. Cycling and running, for example, can give your heart and lungs a good workout, but they won't do much to strengthen your upper body. The same goes for roller skating and aerobic dancing. And though golf, archery and weight training can stretch or strengthen your sinews, they aren't really aerobic. The prime aerobic exercises are rowing, swimming and cross-country skiing, surpassing even such highly rated aerobic activities as walking, volleyball, basketball, hockey, racquetball and jumping rope. And all these vary in their power to give your muscles flexibility and strength.

A sensible strategy is to select a primary aerobic exercise and supplement it if necessary with strengthening and stretching workouts. Experts say that whatever program you select, the aerobic part should get your heart really pumping for 20 minutes or more, at least three times a week.

Did you miss some answers by more than a decade? If so, you know what one gerontologist meant when she said we're becoming an "age-irrelevant society." When you follow a regular program of vigorous exercise, you can be energetic, healthy and trim at any age.

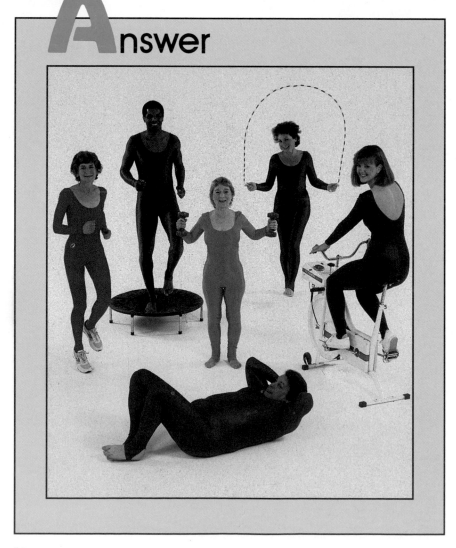

Answer

LOVE IT OR LEAVE IT

Within these guidelines, the makeup of your own program should depend on whether you like it—or whether it likes you. You certainly aren't likely to stick with a workout you hate, no matter how good it is for you. And if it hates you—if it isn't suited to you physically—you could be in for a ton of frustration.

"People who dislike a certain form of exercise probably should never try to persist in it," says Tom Griffin, M.D., an Arizona physician and coauthor of *Feeling Good for Life.* "They're doomed to lose interest fast. And though healthy people can participate in and benefit from almost any kind of workout, a given exercise may be better matched to some people than others."

To help you avoid a mismatch, here's a brief rundown of the physical demands of selected exercises.

Running. This exercise requires high energy output, lots of stamina and a physique free of weaknesses in the knees or spine. And because of its repetitive nature, it's not suited for people who want plenty of variety in their workouts. Serious long-distance running for the aspiring athlete demands good heart/lung power and an ectomorphic (thin and tall) frame with low body weight for height.

Swimming. This is a true "soft exercise" that puts a minimum of stress on muscles and joints. People with excellent heart/lung power, well-developed upper body muscles and a tall, lean frame are naturals at competitive swimming. But if you like long, slow "no-sweat" workouts, swimming is for you.

Cycling. This is soft exercise, too, and perfectly suited for those who want to ease into fitness. It's ideal for large people who want to avoid workouts that put extra strain on their feet and joints. For people whose backs don't take kindly to the vibrations of road cycling, stationary biking is the perfect alternative. Competitive cycling, on the other hand, demands good lung performance and a mesomorphic (average) frame with a narrow front to present to the wind.

Racquetball. Like running, it requires a lot of energy and plenty of endurance. It also demands intense concentration, good hand/eye coordination and moderate agility. Anyone with bad joints or a weak back should probably forgo this fast-moving game. However, it's just the ticket for people who thrive on adrenaline and get bored with running or other monotonous exercises.

Cross-Country Skiing. This exercise requires extensive movement of both legs and arms, making it one of the most aerobically demanding workouts around. Most people need some time to build up enough stamina to comfortably ski the woods and fields. But many people who have achieved a reasonable level of fitness also can enjoy this safe winter activity.

Walking. Experts have hailed walking as the perfect soft exercise—aerobically demanding yet easy on the joints, muscles and heart. To derive physical benefits from it, you need only walk slightly faster than your normal pace, though not so fast that you can't carry on a conversation. Even people with back problems, people with weak joints and people who are overweight can safely walk for fitness.

A FRANK LOOK AT CELLULITE

It's the dimpled and puckered flab that clings to thighs, buttocks, arms and hips—called orange-peel skin by some, cottage-cheese fat by others and cellulite by most. But whatever it's called, cellulite is widely regarded as one of the toughest of all physical blemishes to erase. It's said to afflict eight out of ten women (and a few men) and is the bane of the beauty-conscious.

Popular lore says that cellulite (a term coined in European salons and spas) is not ordinary fat, but "fat gone wrong," a gel-like blend of fat, water and toxins pocketed in tiny lumps just beneath the skin. Press your skin between your hands, some people advise, and you'll proba-

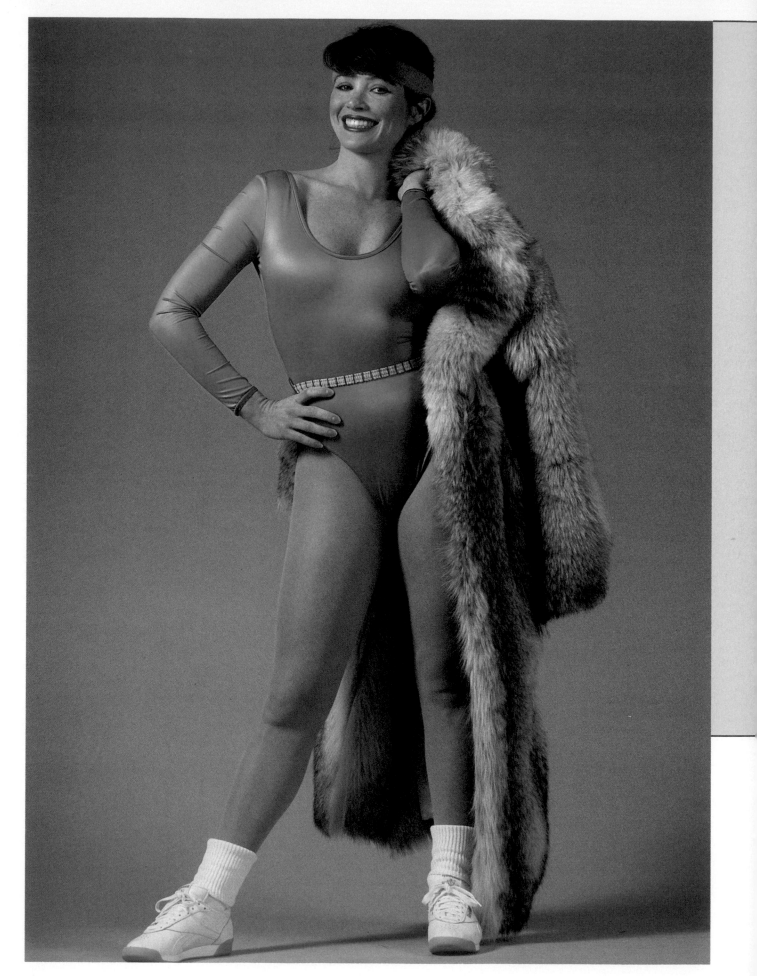

A Fitness Test for Your Workout Clothes

Exercise wear has become high fashion, but the best sports wardrobe combines eye appeal with comfort and safety. Here's what to look for when choosing workout wear that works out for you.

Shoes

They have to be comfortable, of course, but more than that they must be designed for your kind of workout. There are running shoes, court shoes, aerobic shoes and a lot more—and they're not interchangeable.

The right shoe for you also must have the right fit in the heel and toe. It has to hug your heel without chafing it while leaving enough room for you to wiggle your toes. It should give you the proper degree of support and flexibility for your chosen activity. And it must have enough cushioning to protect your foot against impact, but not so much that you lose your sense of contact with the ground.

Warmup Suits

The best of these launder well, maintain their shape, allow your skin to breathe and—of course—keep you warm and dry. Look for those made of 100 percent cotton, a fleece combination of half cotton and half polyester or wind-resistant nylon.

But don't waste your money on rubberized sweat suits. They're supposed to drain fat from your body, but they don't. They can make you sweat off water weight, but the weight comes right back when you eat or drink after working out. And the worst part is that they prevent perspiration from evaporating, thus fouling up your body's cooling system.

Leotards

These give you freedom to stretch and bend—and to look attractive while you're doing it. So leotard rule number one is don't sacrifice this freedom by wearing styles that make you look great standing still but inhibit your movement. Go for the sensible but handsome creations. Try, for example, the alternatives to low-backed leotards that give little or no bust support. They're cut a little higher and have tabs in back to anchor bra straps in place.

Belts

These accessories can define your waist and add dimension to leotards. They come in a myriad of styles and colors, but the only ones worth considering are the elastic ones that stretch when you do. Nonelastic belts (especially the wide, stiff ones) restrict your movement and inhibit your breathing.

Sports Socks

These can help protect your feet from chafing and blisters and absorb shock. The best ones are either cotton or cotton/synthetic blends and have lots of cushioning for heel and sole.

Sports Bras

For most athletic women, sports bras are mandatory equipment. They support and compress the breasts against the chest wall to minimize bounce, reducing wear and tear on the breasts' fibrous tissue. The best designs have nonchafe seams and fasteners, underbands instead of underwires and nonstretch straps to reduce breast movement.

Headbands

These may add panache to your ensemble, but their main job is to keep sweat out of your eyes and sweaty hair off your forehead. So they should be absorbent. The wide cotton-knit bands will do the job. The narrow braided ones won't.

---

bly see the oatmeal lumps of cellulite. For such deformity they blame birth control pills, internal illnesses, environmental pollutants, even—would you believe—miniskirts.

According to a few self-styled experts, getting rid of cellulite is not like getting rid of ordinary fat. Simple dieting and exercise, they say, won't work on this pseudofat. Effective treatment calls for unusual—even bizarre—approaches. Thus the "cures" have included loofah sponges, cactus-fiber washcloths, horsehair mitts, vitamin/mineral supplements, rubberized pants, toning lotions, creams, enzyme injections, vibrating machines and whirlpool baths.

Unfortunately, none of these miracles works. And for good reason. Doctors and researchers point out that cellulite is not "fat gone wrong"—it's just plain fat. Scientists can detect no chemical or structural difference between so-called cellulite fat and common fat. The disorder, therefore, will respond to dieting and exercise, but not to the offbeat remedies that have nothing to do with fat reduction.

Researchers now know that what people call cellulite is simply ordinary fat cells overloaded with fat and bulging underneath the skin in a waffled pattern. "What you see is a combination of fat, poor muscle tone and poor skin tone," says Neil Solomon, M.D., an obesity and weight-control expert in Baltimore. "It's the way the skin fits over whatever fat there is underneath. If a person does not have good muscle tone in an area, say on the thighs, the skin takes on the contours of the fat beneath and appears rippled."

Researchers also know that some people are more prone to the condition than others and the reasons are sex and heredity. A pair of German investigators found that women are more likely than men to have cellulite partly because the fat just beneath women's skin is packed into round fat-cell chambers that can easily bulge underneath the skin, while men's fat-cell chambers are arranged in a more stable design. And perhaps just as important, certain areas of women's skin are actually thinner than men's and have more fat under the surface. Then, too, people vary greatly in their patterns of fat distribution, and children are likely to inherit the patterns of their parents.

But these givens of gender and heredity can be improved upon, and medical professionals say there are only two ways to do it: You have to consistently take in fewer calories than you expend, and you must exercise regularly to tighten up the muscles and make the flabby areas appear taut.

Dr. Solomon emphasizes that in his own studies of weight loss in overweight people with dimpling of the skin on their thighs and buttocks, "those who lost weight lost some of the dimpling."

The German researchers concur with Dr. Solomon and underscore the importance of physical activity in the battle against cellulite. They claim, as other researchers do, that they've seen little or no cellulite among female athletes.

Running, dancing, swimming, cycling—these and other activities can help you burn off flab, but some fitness experts say that one of the best anticellulite exercise is walking. For walking helps pull on—and thus firm—buttocks and thighs, areas most susceptible to "orange-peel skin."

Dr. Solomon does, however, offer a caution to those who try to lose too much too fast: "Don't lose more weight (not more than 5 to 10 pounds a month) than your skin elasticity can keep up with. In an older person, batwing arms and wrinkled, flabby skin on the abdomen are usually the results of too-rapid weight loss and insufficient regular exercise."

Anticellulite Creams

These concoctions may sport French-sounding trade names, contain everything from sea moss to horse chestnuts and boast the power to kill cellulite where it sits. The manufacturers say that the creams can "contour" the body, "tone superficial tissues" and offer "sleekening benefits."

But, alas, the ballyhoo is bunk. A U.S. Food and Drug Administration report points out that despite their exotic contents, the creams include the same types of ingredients as common lubricating lotions: water, emollients, emulsifiers, preservatives, colors and fragrances. And experts have already insisted there isn't a shred of medical evidence that the creams work.

BODY SCULPTING: SLIMMING DOWN THROUGH WEIGHT TRAINING

Sculpt the human body? Carve a new, firmer, trimmer you? It sounds too good to be true, but according to Ralph Carnes, Ph.D., former dean of the College of Arts and Sciences at Roosevelt University in Chicago, it's possible. The secret to body sculpting is working out with weights.

Dr. Carnes, coauthor of *Bodysculpture: Weight Training for Women,* claims that weight training is not just for men who want monumental muscles. It's for men *and* women who want well-toned muscles packed in a shape to be proud of. "You can zero in on your body's trouble spots," he says, "and sculpt a shapelier leg or firm a flabby arm with exercises aimed at those areas."

Weight training, like any exercise, burns calories, and that can mean an overall loss of extra fat. But just as important, lifting weights can enhance muscles in specific areas of the body, giving those areas a firmer and sleeker look. Thus, without losing an ounce, says Dr. Carnes, you can appear to have shaved off pounds.

But is there a danger that weight training will make women look like female versions of Arnold Schwarzenegger? Not really, says Ronald Mackenzie, M.D., medical director of the National Athletic Health Institute in Inglewood, California. "Women normally don't have the amount of male hormones it takes to build bulging muscles," he says. And they have an extra layer of fat that will mute muscle definition and guarantee soft curves, not rugged mountains.

Nor will weight training transform an ectomorph (someone with a tall, thin frame) or an endomorph (someone with a large, heavy frame) into a mesomorph (a person of average build). "You won't change your body type," says Dr. Carnes, "but you will become the best, shapeliest example of the type you have."

(continued on page 103)

Bust Developers: Do They Work?

They may do a great job of boosting the hopes of women who buy them, but not much else. The devices fail because breasts aren't muscles that can be built up like biceps. Breast tissue is mostly glands, ducts and fat. You can develop the muscle around your breasts to firm and lift them, but there's no known apparatus that can manipulate breasts to expand them.

What's more, bust developers recently flunked a scientific test of their effectiveness. In a study at the University of Arizona, 34 women underwent a 21-day breast-expansion program using bust developers. The results: The devices produced absolutely no increase in mammary tissues.

Sculpting Your Body

Body sculpting is a kind of weight training that zeroes in on specific body areas to tone up muscles and slim down bulges. The technique works by reducing overall body fat and firming particular muscles to produce stronger lines. Here are a few body-sculpting exercises, designed by Ralph Carnes, Ph.D., that work on some of your body's most persistent trouble spots.

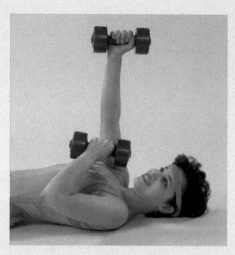

Triceps

Lie on your back on the floor and hold a pair of dumbbells (5 pounds each, or less) directly overhead, arms straight. Then slowly lower the weights toward your chest, bending your elbows. You can work both arms simultaneously or one at a time. Do 10 reps. This tones the triceps (the large muscle on the back of the upper arm) and helps reduce the flabby "batwing" look.

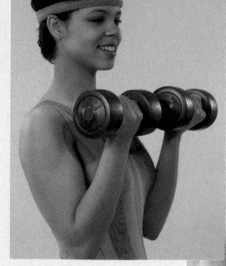

Biceps

Stand erect and hold a dumbbell (5 pounds or less) in each hand, with arms at your sides, palms facing forward. Slowly bend your arms at the elbows and bring the weights up until they touch your chest. Do 10 reps. In women this exercise will tone and define the biceps (the large muscle at the front of the upper arm) but will not excessively enlarge it.

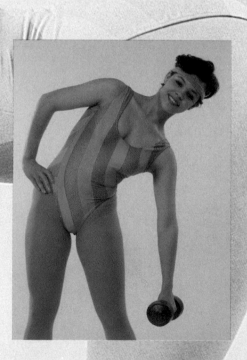

Waist

Stand with arms at your sides with your feet shoulder width apart. Hold a light dumbbell (no more than 5 pounds) in your right hand and slowly bend at the waist to your right side, leaning down as far as you can with legs straight. Then return to erect position. Do 12 to 15 reps, switch to your left side, then do 12 to 15 more.

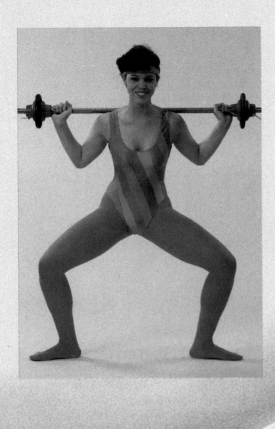

Thighs and Hips

Stand with your feet slightly more than shoulder width apart, with toes angled outward. Hold a barbell across your shoulders and slowly bend your knees until your thighs are parallel to the floor. Then return to the erect position. Do 10 to 12 repetitions, and use enough weight to make the 10th rep a tough one. The exercise gives thigh and hip muscles more definition and—like all body-sculpting exercises—increases blood circulation in the area. Increased circulation is what helps mobilize fat away from those unwanted lumps.

Bust

Lie on your back on the floor and hold a dumbbell weighing 5 pounds or less in each hand. Hold the dumbbells directly over your chest with arms straight, palms facing each other. Then, keeping your arms straight, slowly lower the weights to the floor on each side of you so your body forms a cross. Then bring the weights to the upright position again. Do 10 reps, and gradually work up to 20. This maneuver tones up pectoral muscles (the ones that provide the foundation for the bust) and thus helps to pull breasts up into a more prominent posture.

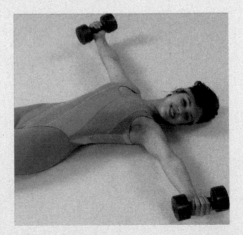

Five Beautifying Posture Tricks

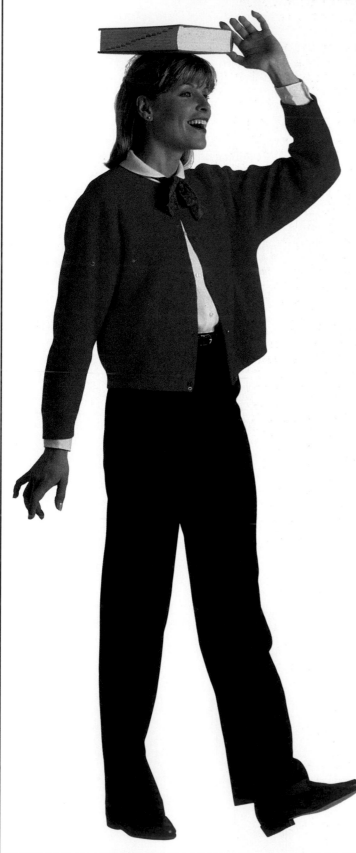

Good posture tips that can radically change your appearance for the better:

• While standing, tilt your lower pelvis forward by contracting the muscles in your buttocks. This simple movement decreases any excess curve in your lower spine, evenly distributing the weight on your back and giving you a more erect and poised look.

• Keep your chin level, straightening your neck into a vertical position. For practice, you can look in a mirror, grasp a tuft of hair from the center of your head and pull up gently, aligning your chin parallel to the floor. Such neck and head adjustments should make you look taller and your neck longer.

• Hold your chest high by relaxing your shoulders and allowing your arms to hang easily at your sides. As you do, your shoulders will automatically pull back where they should be and your bust will appear larger or more prominent. If you're executing the maneuver properly in a standing position, your palms will rotate inward to face your thighs.

• Stand tall. This trick can make you look inches thinner because a shortened stomach muscle, caused by slumping, makes you appear paunchy. It's the aesthetic complement—and to some extent the natural result—of raising your chest.

• Stand with your feet parallel, not with your toes pointed outward, with your weight evenly distributed between the front and back of your feet. If you're standing properly, you shouldn't be able to see your heels when you look at your feet in a mirror. The stance enables you to maintain the erect and graceful posture you want. In the toes-outward position your knees lock and your lower pelvis is tilted backward— the prelude to a slumped posture.

In the process, you will enjoy weight training's most celebrated advantage: increased strength and stamina. And the by-product of these is a decreased risk of health problems caused in part by weak muscles—back strain, hernia, joint troubles and poor posture. James Skinner, Ph.D., professor of physical education at Arizona State University, believes that the strengthening brought about by weight training can even benefit you in sports. "If you work on your arms and shoulders," he says, "you'll have fewer problems with tennis elbow, you'll hit the ball harder and you'll be able to play longer."

The whole idea of weight training, of course, is to make your muscles work harder against resistance. But what do you use to get that resistance, free weights or machines like Nautilus or Universal? In terms of effect on your looks, says Dr. Carnes, both approaches are good, but working with free weights has an added advantage—this approach strengthens the muscles that stabilize your joints. Not only is this exercise good for your joints, it also makes you look sleeker.

But no matter what kind of resistance you select, you have to follow instructions and use common sense. Go slowly, try not to overdo it and keep the following points in mind.

- Using lighter weights to perform 10 to 20 repetitions will firm muscles and increase endurance. Using heavier weights with 8 repetitions will build muscle size and strength.

- For an effective workout you have to select weights that will let you raise a good sweat in 8 to 15 repetitions.

- A beginner's routine would include 8 to 15 repetitions of basic exercises that work every part of your body, from leg curls for your thighs to bench presses for your shoulders and arms. Workouts should be 40 to 60 minutes long, done two or three times a week. As you improve, you need to increase the size of the weights and the intensity and frequency of your routines to continue producing results.

- If you're going to use a gym, you must choose it carefully. It should have all the equipment you need, and the staff should be able to show you how to use each piece of equipment and help you plan an individual program—one that's built around *your* needs and proceeds at *your* pace.

- You should be in good general health to start a weight training program. And it's a good idea to inform your doctor of your exercise plans.

Seven Ways to Relax

Can you ever really look your best when you're tense, nervous or stressed? Certainly not. So here is a variety of simple but effective relaxation techniques that can calm you down, perk you up or just plain make you feel—and look—brand new.

1 Give Yourself a Feel-Good Foot Massage

What part of you deserves TLC more than your feet? After all, they take an awful pounding every day. And when they kick up a fuss, it's tough—some people say impossible—to look your best.

Start your foot massage by applying pressure with your thumbs to the soles, making sure to cover every square inch. Do the same to the rest of your feet, giving special attention to the parts that hurt. Be sure to devote some time to your Achilles tendons. And after pressing on your toes, move them from side to side and bend them gently forward and backward.

3 Calm Yourself with Color

Think of your favorite color, then relax the muscles in your neck and shoulders. If you repeat this simple exercise a few times a day for several weeks, you'll find that when you think of the color, your neck and shoulder muscles will automatically relax, without any conscious effort on your part. And after you have one color working for your body, you can associate other colors with other muscle groups. You thus could have a whole rainbow of hues helping you to overcome tension.

2 Breathe a Little Easier

When you're overwrought or under severe stress, your breathing is rapid and shallow. But slow down and deepen your breathing and you can actually reverse the effects of overstress. So say a number of experts, including Jenny Steinmetz, Ph.D., a psychologist at the Kaiser Permanente Medical Center in Hayward, California.

"I tell my clients to slow their breathing to a 7-second inhale and an 8-second exhale," she says. "Do 4 of those per minute for a total of 2 minutes, and that discharges the stress immediately."

4 Use the Power of PR

Progressive Relaxation (PR) is a proven technique for vanquishing physical and mental tension. First, lie down and close your eyes. Then make a tight fist with your right hand, tensing the muscles in your wrist and forearm. Hold for 5 seconds, feeling the tension, then unclench and let the tension drain from your forearm, wrist and fingers. Note the difference between the feeling of tautness and the pleasure of total relaxation. Now repeat this tension/relaxation sequence for your left hand, then for your upper arms, shoulders, neck, face, legs, feet and toes. Once you master it, you can practice it anywhere, anytime—in a traffic jam, before the big board meeting or in any other situation that makes you tense.

5 Take a Mental Vacation

Following Progressive Relaxation, try another technique, called visualization. Together the techniques require about 20 minutes of your time. Sit back in your easy chair, close your eyes and take 5 minutes to recall the sights and sounds of a tranquil moment from your past: a running brook, a snow-covered hillside, a pastel sunset, whatever appeals to you. You may come back from the trip a new person.

6 Say the Magic Word

Try a simple, relaxing form of meditation. Close your eyes and slowly repeat the same word over and over again, preferably a word ending in "m" or "n" like "home," "ocean" or "calm." The exercise, some experts say, helps quiet the central nervous system and counters the stress response.

7 Stretch the Tension Away

Stretching is more than just a prelude to vigorous exercise. It's an incredibly effective way to relax. For best results, do a slow, sustained stretch of specific muscles, creating only mild tension in them, for 10 to 30 seconds. For example, try standing on your toes, extending your arms toward the ceiling. Or bending over while sitting, touching your toes. Or clasping your hands behind your head, drawing your head gently down toward your chest.

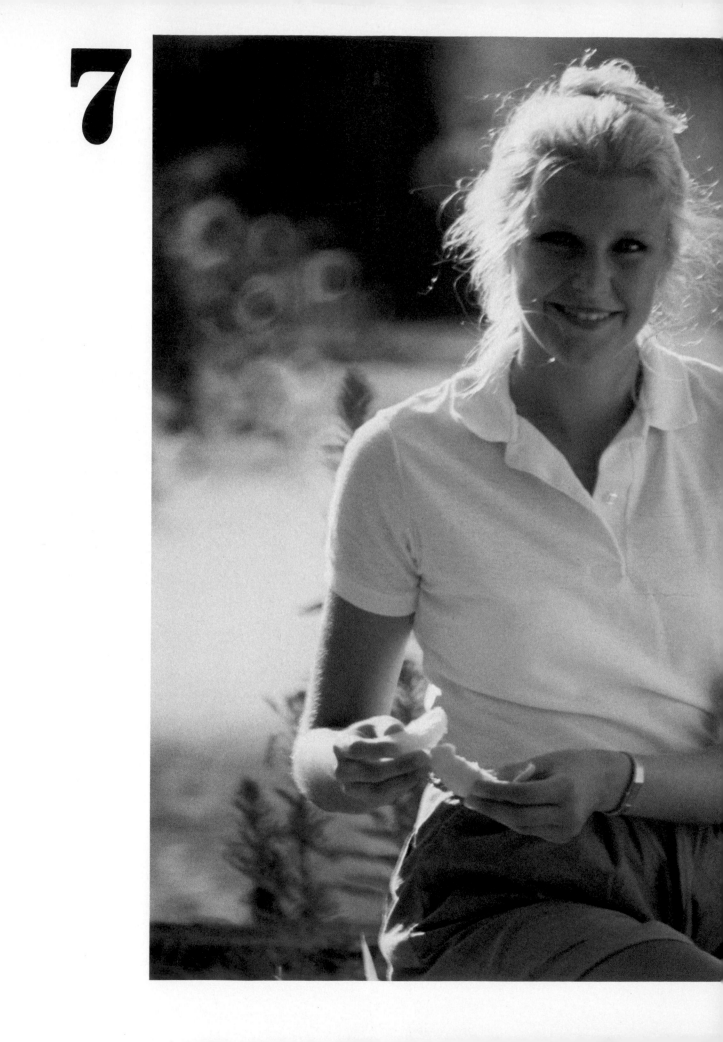

7

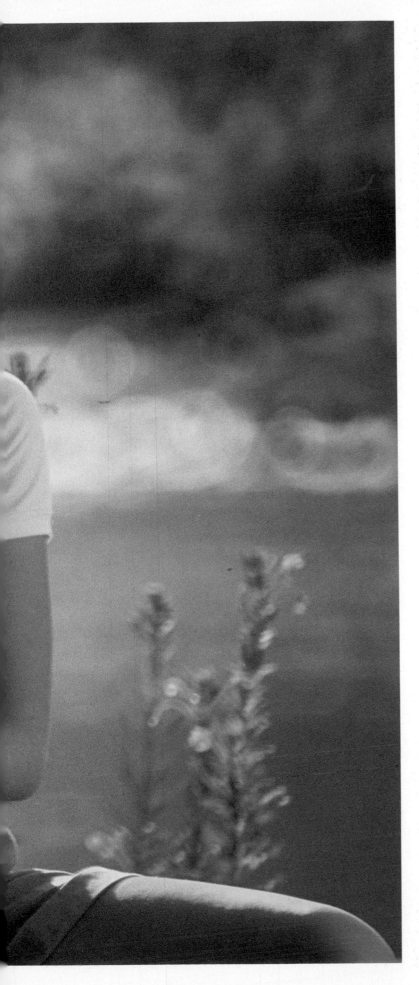

Nurturing Your Beauty

Discover the key nutrients that build beauty from the inside out.

Most people have heard that eating oranges and other citrus fruit can help to fight colds. As you digest an orange, vitamin C is released to fight infection. *Wearing* an orange slice to try to get the same effect would be silly. Yet that's just about what we do when we try to improve our skin and hair by using beauty care products that claim to coat us with a healing mix of protein, wheat germ or some other nutrient-rich ingredient. Not that these products aren't on the right track— nutrients are crucial to your appearance. But it's the nutrients we put *in* us, not *on* us, that really count. A healthy diet— fresh food with lots of vitamins and minerals and fiber, low in fat, sugar and salt—is the only sure way to nourish your skin and hair.

In fact, the connection between what you eat and how you look is quite direct. Consider what happens when you don't get enough nutrients. A few months of consuming too little iron, for example, can leave you with brittle nails, thin hair and pale lips and skin. No amount of nail polish, conditioner or lipstick can duplicate the glow that comes from iron-rich blood. Similarly, a short supply of riboflavin (vitamin B_2), can lead to oily hair, flaky patches around the hairline, eyebrows and nose, cracks at the corners of your mouth or red, inflamed eyelids. White spots on your fingernails could mean that you aren't getting enough zinc.

That's what happens when you're short-changed. The other side of the coin is the good things that happen when you get your fair share of certain nutrients. Like vitamin A.

Vitamin A is nature's makeup: It gives cantaloupes, sweet potatoes and green peppers their gorgeous hues. (In fact, it's found abundantly in most dark green, yellow or red fruits and vegetables.) So perhaps it's no accident that a

Water: Your Skin's Primary Nutrient

Your skin depends on water to remain soft and smooth. When water reaches 10 percent or more of your skin's weight, it makes your skin look great—firm, supple and clear. Any less water and your skin begins to feel dry and flaky.

To hydrate from within, you need the equivalent of 8 glasses of water a day. Here's how to help get your daily quota.

- Spike your beverages—fruit juice and so on—with plain or seltzer water.
- Drink plain ice water with every meal.
- Eat plenty of juicy fruits and vegetables, such as berries, melons, tomatoes, peaches and asparagus, which are at least 80 percent water by weight.

person's "covering" needs vitamin A, too. A-rich foods act like a facial from the inside out because the vitamin is essential to the health of the cells that keep skin smooth and resilient. And because hair and nails grow from your skin, what's good for your skin is equally good for its accessories.

PROTEIN POWER

Your hair is strands of protein. Your nails are small shields of protein. Collagen—the cellular cement that keeps skin firm—is protein. No wonder this nutrient has long been part of the beauty mystique. And no wonder that crash dieting—which starves skin, hair and nails of this primary ingredient—takes a toll on your appearance. Your skin will look pale and saggy, and your nails will break as easily as eggshells. Your hair may begin to fall out, too. Starving yourself to stay thin prompts your body to conserve protein by shifting growing hairs into their resting phase, speeding their natural demise. And since protein-starved hair loses its resilience, it falls out easily when you comb or brush it.

In your efforts to pack enough protein into your diet, take care not to load up on fat. The following foods are protein-rich and also fairly low in fat: lean meats, chicken, fish, skim milk or low-fat yogurt. You can also fill your protein requirements by combining beans (or any soy product) and whole grains in the same meal. This gives you enough of the essential amino acids, the chemical building blocks that link up in your body to form protein. Nuts and seeds also fill the protein bill—but they may fill your calorie quota rather quickly, too.

How about the purported power of unflavored gelatin—protein derived from animal "by-products"—to strengthen brittle nails? There's no reason why any other source of protein couldn't do the job equally well if not better, especially since gelatin isn't a top-notch form of protein, lacking one of the nine essential amino acids. Besides, reports on gelatin's nail-strengthening powers are conflicting and unscientific. But if you decide to give gelatin a

try, don't expect to see any results for at least five or six months, if at all. And beware of gelatin desserts that contain sugar and corn syrup. While they might do your nails some good, they're certain to be tough on your teeth.

A NUTRITION PLAN FOR TERRIFIC TEETH

Whenever you eat sugar of any kind—white, brown, honey, molasses, or even the natural sugar in apples and other wholesome foods—the sweet stuff feeds the bacteria on your teeth that in turn produce acids that can dissolve tooth enamel. Tooth enamel may be the hardest substance in your body, but it's no match for these sugar-fueled microbes. The result? Cavities.

Now you know and we know that sugar is here to stay. For one thing, it's in wholesome foods like fruit. For another, that occasional cheesecake or sundae has a way of creeping onto the menu no matter how careful we are. So, while you should try to cut back on sugar if your sweet tooth is overactive, here are a few ways to have your cake—and eat it with beautiful teeth, too.

- Sugar eaten *with* meals is less destructive than sugar eaten *alone*. You secrete more saliva with meals, which helps neutralize destructive acids and quickly clears sugar from your mouth. On the other hand, sugary snacks do the most damage when eaten at bedtime, when saliva flow is the lowest.
- Not all sweets are created equal. The worst—at least as far as your teeth are concerned—are sticky foods like fudge, jelly, jam, jelly beans, syrups, caramels, toffee, marshmallows and dried fruit. These sweets tend to cling to your teeth, prolonging acid production and prompting decay. Similarly, acid production remains in high gear while you suck on slow-dissolving lozenges or cough drops.
- Cheese, carrots and bananas have special decay-resistant properties all their own. Researchers at the National Insti-

tute of Dental Research found that cheese reduces acid production, and carrots and bananas prompt bacteria to clump together so that they're easier to brush away. Use them for between-meal or late-night snacks.

DRINKS THAT DRY OUT YOUR SKIN

Sugary drinks pack a double whammy: not only do they bathe your teeth in sweets, but they can dehydrate you because your body has to draw water from the cells to dilute the sugar. Beverages containing caffeine and alcohol can also drain you; they stimulate the kidneys to work overtime.

This diuretic effect of soft drinks, coffee, tea and alcohol probably comes as no surprise to regular imbibers. Most know all too well their power to necessitate frequent trips to the restroom. And hangover veterans know that too much alcohol can leave your mouth feeling as though it's lined with sandpaper. What you may not realize is that diuretic beverages can leave your skin and lips dry and parched, too.

Just how much alcohol, for example, do you have to drink before your skin begins to look reptilian? Few experts are willing to venture a guess at the precise amount of alcohol that can leave you high *and* dry. But if you indulge as though every Saturday night is New Year's Eve, your skin will eventually show it: not only will it be dry, but tiny wrinkles will be more noticeable. So if you get a kick out of champagne—or any other alcoholic beverage—go easy. Drink plenty of water when you do drink alcohol, and spike your spirits with seltzer water to make up for lost fluids.

If your problem isn't too little but too *much* water in your body—water retention that shows up as puffy eyes or swollen ankles—a dietary change may again be the solution: less salt. Biochemically, salt helps maintain the pressure inside the cells; add more salt and the body has to retain water to keep things balanced. Subtract salt and the excess water will probably go with it.

LITTLE MISS MUFFET VS THE INCREDIBLE SHRINKING WOMAN

Little Miss Muffet sat on a tuffet eating her curds and whey. And thanks to her curds and whey, she sat very straight and tall.

Milk products (curd and whey portions alike) supply plenty of calcium, the mineral primarily responsible for strong, healthy bones. Without enough calcium, women past menopause succumb to osteoporosis, or thin, brittle bones. As a result, their backbones collapse, leaving them stooped, frail and up to 3 inches shorter than they were in their 20s.

You can buy all the designer clothes you can afford, but if you don't stand straight and tall, you won't look your best. Yet of all the beauty-enhancing vitamins and minerals, calcium can be the most difficult to obtain through diet alone. The richest food sources—milk and cheese—are relatively high in fat and calories, making quantities large enough to fulfill calcium requirements off-limits to people who watch their weight. And adults usually have far less lactase (the enzyme that digests lactose, or milk sugar) than they did as children, making milk difficult to digest.

To help maintain a statuesque physique and youthful stride throughout life, women past 35 can—and should—rely on calcium supplements. Calcium carbonate contains 40 percent calcium—400 milligrams per 1,000-milligram tablet—making it one of the richest sources of calcium around. Three tablets a day supply as much calcium as a quart of milk. That's all you need to maintain the stature and strength that healthy bones alone can provide.

In order to assimilate as much calcium as possible, take calcium at bedtime so your system can absorb the mineral and shuttle it to your bones with no interference from protein or other dietary influences.

A Guide to Beauty Nutrients

Your local supermarket stocks as many "beauty products" as a department store cosmetics counter. These include beautifying agents like whole grains, fresh fruits and vegetables, yogurt, lean meat, chicken, fish and other foods listed in the following guide. Certain key nutrients supplied by those foods are indispensable to healthy-looking skin, hair and nails and strong teeth and bones.

In addition to the vitamins and minerals featured here, remember that fiber—the indigestible framework of fruits, vegetables, legumes and whole grains—is considered important to the prevention of varicose veins.

Dieters need to pay particular attention to their shopping list: Everything that you plunk into your grocery cart should be chock-full of vitamins and minerals to avoid shortchanging yourself nutritionally.

vitamin A

From: Beef liver, sweet potatoes, carrots, spinach, cantaloupe and other green, yellow and orange fruits and vegetables

Can Help to: Keep skin soft and supple; prevent dry, flaky skin; build strong bones by fostering reproduction of bone cells.

IRON

From: Beef liver, lean beef, blackstrap molasses, sunflower seeds, chickpeas, dark meat of poultry (best eaten with a rich source of vitamin C to boost iron absorption)

Can Help to: Prevent anemia, which leads to brittle nails, hair loss, pale lips and skin.

vitamin E

From: Wheat germ and wheat germ oil, sunflower seeds and oil, almonds, pecans, hazelnuts and other nuts

Can Help to: Heal dry, rough, red skin; protect skin against damaging effects of sunburn; prevent dry hair; slow down cellular aging at all levels.

(Shortage of vitamin E may cause yellow nails.)

vitamin D

From: Sunshine, vitamin-D-fortified milk, fish-liver oil, herring, mackerel, salmon, tuna

Can Help to: Build strong bones.

B vitamins

From: Whole grains, poultry, legumes, green leafy vegetables, brewer's yeast

Can Help to: Provide sufficient folate, which teams up with other nutrients to protect against receding or bleeding gums. (Too little vitamin B_{12} can cause darkened nails.)

CALCIUM

From: Skim milk, yogurt, cheese, salmon (with bones), tofu, broccoli, calcium carbonate supplements

Can Help to: Build strong bones; prevent rounded shoulders and ensure straight posture, preserving a youthful stride; protect against tooth decay and gum recession.

PROTEIN

From: Lean meat, chicken, fish, skim milk and cheese, tofu, combinations of beans, seeds, nuts and grains

Can Help to: Maintain firm, smooth, glowing skin, strong hair and nails.

C

From: Citrus juice, cantaloupe, peppers, strawberries, potatoes and other fresh fruits and vegetables

Can Help to: Keep joints lubricated; guard against infection; build strong bones by facilitating absorption of calcium and iron; keep gums firm and pink; heal cold sores (especially when taken with bioflavonoids, also found in citrus fruits and fresh vegetables).

ZINC

From: Lean beef, lamb, liver (chicken, beef or calves'), turkey, pumpkin seeds, various legumes

Can Help to: Maintain healthy hair and scalp; keep complexion clear; strengthen fingernails; fight body odor; aid calcium in the prevention of weak, brittle bones and poor posture from osteoporosis.

8

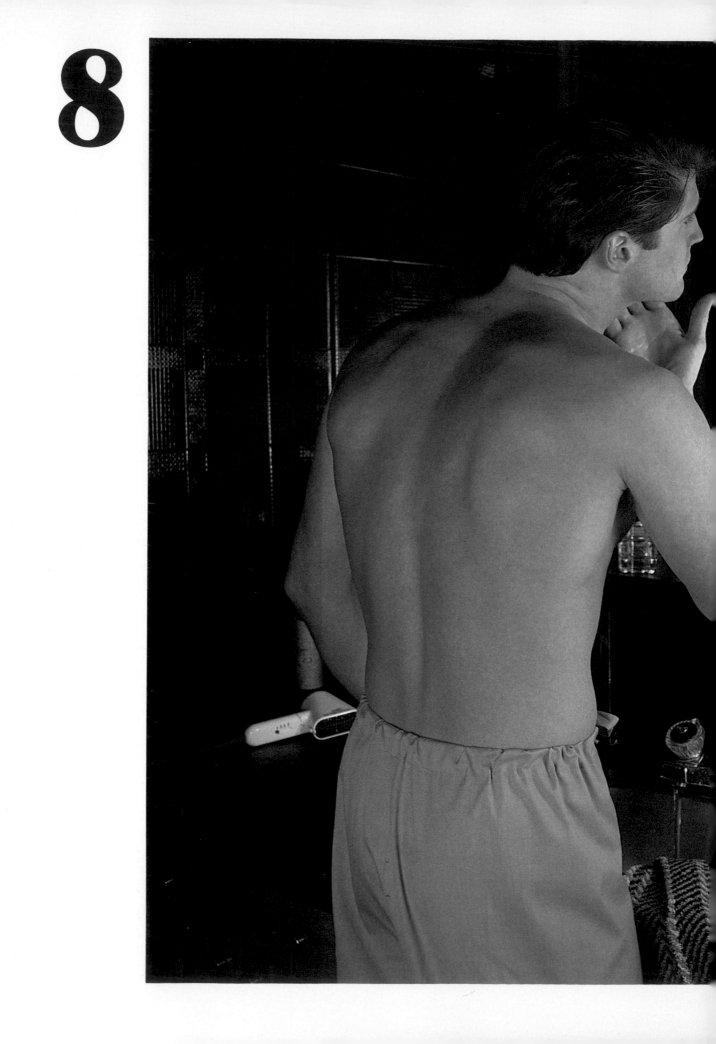

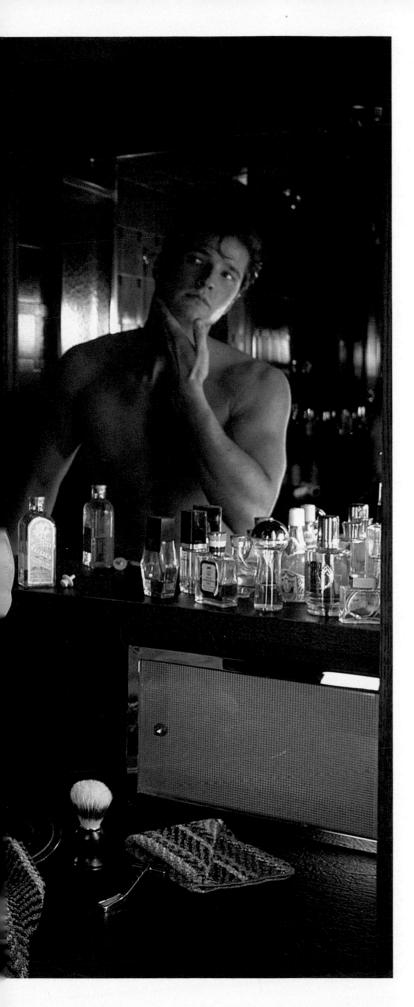

For the Well-Groomed Man

A no-nonsense guide to improving your looks, updating your style.

Men are caught in an odd kind of bind. While no one bats an eyelash at the sight of a woman primping in public, a man is supposed to be supremely uninterested in the whole business of good grooming. He's supposed to look good—but without caring about it. It's considered a woman's right—even *duty*—to devote time, trouble and money to the task of enhancing her own beauty, but men, for the most part, are confined to the sidelong glance in the shopping mall mirror.

The truth, of course, is that men *do* care about their looks, and always have. They're as concerned about preserving their youthfulness and putting their best face forward as anyone else. Yet (perhaps partly because of the social taboo against appearing to care *too much*) until recently men have remained relatively uninformed about the basics of hair and skin care.

All that's changing, though—and fast. Today, on the heels of the health and fitness revolution, there's been among men a renaissance of interest in things that were once the mysterious and sacred province of women. "Ten years ago, when a man came to see me about his skin, he always had an excuse," says men's skin care specialist Lia Schorr, who operates a salon in New York City. "They'd say, 'my wife sent me, or my girlfriend did, or my mother.' Now they don't make excuses anymore. They've taken the responsibility for looking good on themselves."

Men's new openness about trying to look their best hasn't gone unnoticed by the cosmetics companies, either. Marketers have begun hungrily circling the male ego, and department store cosmetics counters have sprouted grooming products "for men" by the score—from moisturizers to astringents, from "bronzers" to shaving creams for three types of skin.

It doesn't have to cost a lot to look your best. But it does take a little learning, a splash of style—and a solid foundation of good health.

MEN'S SKIN CARE

Few men have any interest in keeping their skin as white and tender as a poached chicken. And why should they? Real men are supposed to be tough as cowhide, with skin to prove it. At least, that's the gospel according to Madison Avenue (when it's selling something other than skin care products). Unfortunately, the truth is that the modern urban male who neglects his skin will tend to end up looking not so much ruggedly windburned as just plain old and tired.

One of the most common results of neglect is dry skin, a condition dermatologists call xerosis. Americans spend a half billion dollars a year on products for this one skin problem alone. The basic plan of attack on dry, chapped skin is this: You've got to raise your skin's moisture level and keep it there at the same time you prevent water from escaping across its surface.

Dermatologist Kenneth Arndt, M.D., writing in *The Harvard Medical School Health Letter Book,* suggests that "the most effective means to correct dryness and add protection is to soak the dry area in water for 5 to 10 minutes, then apply a greasy ointment such as petrolatum (Vaseline) or lanolin, or somewhat lighter preparations," like Keri,

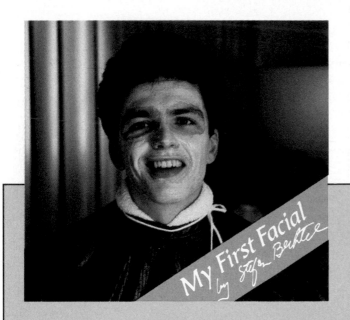

My First Facial by Stefan Bechtel

Like most men, I would make an appointment for a facial about as soon as I'd make one for a facelift. But my assignment was to satisfy your curiosity (and my own). So, feeling a little foolish, I walked into Lia Schorr's salon on Madison Avenue in New York to give it a try.

Ms. Schorr, a dark-haired Israeli beauty, began by applying a massage cream to my face, neck and shoulders with swift repeating strokes. She explained that the point of a facial was to give the skin the sort of really deep cleansing, nourishment and stimulation that's beyond even a conscientious daily skin care program. And, of course, "to pamper the client—and men love that more than anyone."

Next she laid a cloth over my eyes and directed a steady blast of hot steam onto my face to open and disinfect the pores. Then, under a bright, close light, she worked over my pores with tissue-wrapped fingertips, squeezing them free of clogged-up dirt and oil. Then came a clay-based cleansing mask, which "set" in 10 minutes, drawing my skin taut. Lia rinsed this off and applied the final, "light peeling" mask, which dried like shrinkwrap plastic and took off the outer layer of dead cells when she removed it.

And that was that. It took about an hour and cost $34. My skin tingled, my whole body felt relaxed—but I still don't look like Paul Newman.

Lubriderm or Nivea cream. Dr. Arndt adds: "A person may need to experiment to find the product that works best; products with fancy names, high prices and exotic ingredients are no more effective than others." Since these products don't *add* moisture so much as seal it in, they're best applied when your skin is damp.

Overzealous use of soap also can dry out your skin. That's because soap cleanses your skin of oil and dirt by dissolving or "emulsifying" them—but the detergents and alkaline agents that do this trick also strip the skin of natural, protective oils. Which soaps are best? A 1979 study in the *Journal of the American Academy of Dermatology* showed that among 18 well-known toilet soaps, Dove was by far the mildest.

Another thing to avoid is bathing too often, especially in hot water. Like harsh soap, hot water strips the skin of sebum and tends to hasten drying. Because dry skin tends to itch, your inclination may be to actually *increase* the number of showers and baths you take in an attempt to "wash it off"; instead, bathe less and you're bound to itch less. And when you *do* treat yourself to a warm soak, some dermatologists recommend adding a little bath oil to the water to help seal in moisture by coating the skin (products like Alpha-Keri, Domol or Lubath work well).

Other common causes of dry skin: Overexposure to drying solvents, disinfectants and chemicals (track down the offender and avoid it); overexposure to sun; dry air (protect your hands with gloves in winter, and use humidifiers indoors); and skin diseases like psoriasis, eczema or ichthyosis (get the disease diagnosed and treated).

DON'T BE RASH

Besides overdrying your skin, heavy-handed soap use can also sometimes lead to rashes and fungus infections—even though you thought getting rid of them was part of the point of soap! Soap is mildly antibacterial, it's true—but not all bacteria are bad. "If you scrub yourself excessively with soap, you can permanently deplete certain benign strains of skin bacteria, which can be replaced by less desirable ones that cause skin problems: rashes, impetigo and fungus infections," explains New York dermatologist Dr. Jonathan Zizmor.

Other skin infections and rashes like folliculitis (a bacterial infection

Basic Care for Your Hands

Your hands are the most ingenious and useful of all tools—yet they still "don't get no respect." You act out your whole life with your hands, whether you're fixing a carburetor or signing a contract. Yet most men rarely even notice their hands until they've gotten so cracked and dry they've actually started to bleed, or a strange rash gets completely out of control.

Well, that's just dumb—and it's not very healthy, either. Cracked skin is an open invitation to infection, and an untended rash may spread. It pays to pay your hands some respect.

- First, be aware of your hands by noticing when they've become dry and chapped, or the cuticles are splitting, or you're getting a rash.
- To head off scaling, cracking and chapping—especially if you've got naturally dry skin—find a hand cream you like and use it regularly. Vaseline Intensive Care Lotion, Nivea cream or (much pricier) Serious Hand Cream, from Aramis, should do the trick. But since most commercial lotions work fine, the important thing is not so much which one you use as how often you use it.
- If you work with solvents, disinfectants, waxes or other chemicals, protect your hands with waterproof gloves. Protect them from dry winter air with wool-lined leather gloves.
- It's best not to trim hard, cracked cuticles because that can infect the nail and encourage thicker growth. Instead, keep them soft by massaging cuticle cream or lotion into the nail area or soaking your fingertips in warm water with a dollop of bath oil in it. Then *gently* push back the cuticle with a fingertip or an orange stick wrapped in cotton.
- Too much sun will age the skin on your hands as fast as skin anywhere else— faster, in fact, because hands are exposed so much of the time. So use a sunscreen outdoors or a combination moisturizer/sunscreen to prevent liver spots and dryness.

Grooming Products Guide

Men are becoming very sophisticated from the neck up," a cosmetics buyer from Bloomingdale's told the *Wall Street Journal*. "They no longer just use Colgate and throw on aftershave." Still, the number of grooming products competing for men's attention—many of them marketed specifically for men—has many a male bewildered. What are they all for? Which ones really work? What's the best buy? (One clue: "For men" often means simply "higher priced.") Here's a thumbnail guide.

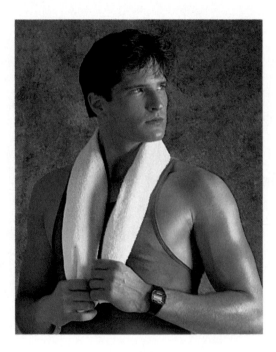

Astringents

For use *only* by men with oily skin, astringents are designed to strip your face of oil and grease while they give your skin a pleasant, tingling kick. Most are mainly plain old witch hazel and rubbing alcohol. If you're after something fancier, try some of the products marketed as "skin toners."

Antiwrinkle Products

Believe it or not, these preparations actually do work—for a little while. They work their brief magic by smoothing and softening your skin with oils and "erasing" wrinkles by causing the skin to swell up slightly due to mild irritation. You may look younger, if only for one night. Try Clinique's Wrinkle Stick or Revlon's Moon Drops Eye Wrinkle Stick.

Antiperspirants

The critical ingredient in all antiperspirants is an astringent salt, usually an aluminum salt, which reduces the flow of sweat up to 55 percent. Antiperspirants also reduce odor by killing bacteria. Your best bet is a product containing aluminum chlorohydrate, which is least likely to irritate your skin or stain your clothes.

of the hair follicles) may respond to topical ointments like bacitracin, an antibiotic, or antiseptics like Betadine or Efudine. Nasty, itching rashes caused by fungal infections (like athlete's foot or "jock itch") take a more holistic approach. To make life miserable for the fungus, which loves dampness, dry thoroughly after bathing, powder with cornstarch and wear absorbent clothing and sandals when you can get away with it. Then blast it with effective, nonprescription medicines: tolnaftate (found in products such as Tinactin), or undecylenic acid (found in products such as Desenex).

Fitness enthusiasts may develop their own special skin problems, like "bikini bottom," annoying wet blisters on the buttocks caused by staying wet for hours. Swimmers and hot tubbers are good candidates for this one. "Wrestler's herpes"—sometimes due to the sexually transmitted form of the virus—can sometimes get passed around among athletes in contact sports. But the most common sports-related skin problem—sun exposure—is the easiest to treat. Outdoor athletes should generously apply sunscreens or sunblocks before heading off to battle and not neglect the easily forgotten places like the back of the neck and the ears.

HAIR: TOPPING IT ALL OFF

It used to be so simple. Saturday mornings, men went down to the barber shop to read dog-eared hunt-

Bronzers

These products give you a "fake" tan. That is, they contain a coal tar derivative called dihydroxy acetone that dyes your skin an orangey-brown. Though they're safe to use, they tend to look fake unless supplemented with a little *real* tan, and they can discolor hair and clothing.

Buf · Puf

Dermatologists call it epibrasion and all it means is vigorous scrubbing to remove dead skin cells, dirt and oil from the skin surface. It feels good, makes you look good and it's healthy—if you don't scrub too hard. This little item, the Buf·Puf, is specially made for that purpose.

Concealers

Yep, they're cosmetics for men. A touch of this little stick (Erace, by Max Factor) will help cover up minor imperfections like dark shadows under the eyes or liver spots. They're usually made of mineral oil or lanolin, talc, a covering agent like zinc oxide, and beeswax.

Deodorants

These products kill odor by killing bacteria; they don't reduce wetness. So if odor is more of a problem for you than wetness, pick a deodorant rather than an antiperspirant. Most people are able to clear up odor problems simply by bathing regularly—and if you don't have a problem, why use a deodorant or antiperspirant at all?

Dry Skin Soap

Soaps for men with dry, flaky skin are "superfatted," meaning they've got extra fats and oils in them to help seal in your skin's moisture. A convenient choice is Softsoap, a mild detergent in a dispenser, or Tone, Dove or Caress.

Moisturizers

Oil of Olay? But isn't that for women? Sure—but some of the best, least expensive moisturizers marketed for women work just as well for men. All moisturizers are basically just oil-based formulas designed to hold moisture in your skin.

Petroleum Jelly

Vaseline? Isn't that for babies' bums? Yes—but it's also the cheapest, most widely available, most effective moisturizer around. Pure petroleum jelly provides your skin with an optimal protective coating. The trick: Use it sparingly, rubbing a little dab into your skin until it disappears.

Shampoos

Shampoos marketed "for men" are almost invariably more expensive, even though there's no real difference between a man's hair and a woman's hair. The main thing is to shop around for a shampoo you like. "Men are very old-fashioned," says beautician Lia Schorr. "They'll use the same product for years, even if it doesn't work for them." Dare to change!

Sunscreens

Nothing ages your skin faster than too many perfect tans. Especially at the beginning of summer, pick a sunscreen with a high Sun Protection Factor (SPF)—15 is the highest you'll need—and PABA, the most effective sun protection agent around. Some moisturizers also have sunscreens built in.

---

ing magazines, swap sports predictions and "get their ears lowered," quick, cheap and easy. A woman never set foot in a barber shop unless chaperoning a small boy. Instead, the "beauty salon" was her private province, where she went to gossip, have her nails done and sit for hours with a UFO on her head. Or something. (To men, it was never quite clear what went on there.)

Today, along with everything else, good grooming has become a bit more complicated. The sexual distinctions have become increasingly blurred. Many hair stylists today number as many men as women among their customers. Plenty of men use blow dryers and styling gels like pros. Some even go so far as to get professional body waves, color or highlights in their hair.

"Men are *much* more style-conscious than they were, say, ten years ago," says Francisco, a hair stylist at Vidal Sassoon's New York salon. "Men feel more comfortable asking for something like a perm, where not so long ago they'd feel like a sissy or something. The point is this: They've recognized how much better they can look. People compliment them. They feel better about themselves. And that's what's made them more open to things that were once considered strictly for women."

The plain fact is that a professional stylist or beautician can usually do a lot more for you than a down-home barber (as well they should, if their prices match their skills).

For instance, says Francisco, "I'll try to show a man how manipulating his hair this way or that will accentuate a certain feature, or downplay another. Given his facial features, I'll try to demonstrate the various style options I think he's got."

More than likely, a stylist has a far better notion than you do about all the things you *could* do. A man who is disturbed by the ever-widening swath of gray around his temples but who also resists the idea of dyeing his whole head could compromise with "lowlights"—that is, breaking up the field of gray with thin streaks of hair colored the natural color of the rest of his hair. Men with lusterless hair can brighten it up and bring out the hidden color more vividly by using temporary color conditioners. Men concerned about a noticeably receding hairline can have their hair slightly lightened or darkened to match their skin tone more closely, so the hairline becomes less visible. In short, men are now party to those strange, secret things women have been doing all these years.

Despite the new openness about looking good, though, many men are still resistant to the notion of patronizing a "beauty salon." Old habits, like old soldiers, don't die without a fight. For that reason, many salons have a separate cutting and styling area for men. "Men like an atmosphere that's informal, simple, and not too prissy, without a lot of women bustling around," says beautician Lia Schorr. The New Age man can get first-class service for his looks—and *still* read dog-eared hunting magazines in peace.

Men are also resistant to the seductions of styling salons because of that age-old double standard governing male beauty: You're supposed to look good, but you're not supposed to fuss with your looks. Says Michel Obadia, co-owner of the chic New York hair salon Pierre Michel: "There's a lot of art and subtlety in men's hair styling, because you're trying to make your client look good—without letting anybody

What to Do for Shaving Nicks

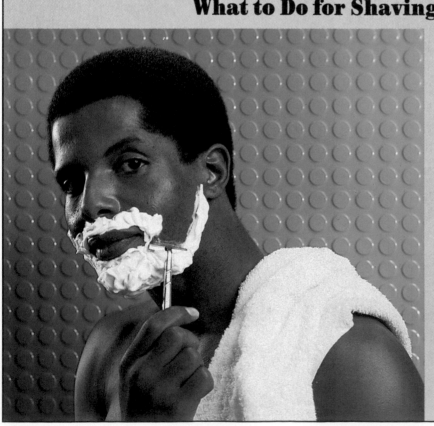

For the man with an unsteady hand, nicks and cuts are a constant problem. Solution: The styptic pencil, which will stop the bleeding almost immediately with a single touch, costs almost nothing and should last a lifetime. The active ingredient is usually aluminum sulfate, which acts as an astringent to close up bleeding vessels (it's the same stuff used in antiperspirants to close perspiring pores). Ordinary alum also works. You can mix up your own styptic lotion using alum, glycerin and water. Or, simplest of all, just step into a cold shower.

know what's going on. Nobody likes a man who always seems to be gazing at his own reflection. You're supposed to look at him and notice how good his skin looks, how youthful he seems, how flattering his hairstyle is, but not have the sense he just walked out of a salon or that his looks are uppermost in his mind."

IS YOUR HAIRSTYLE UP-TO-DATE?

Usually, says Francisco, it's the women—wives, girlfriends, aunts, mothers—who first suggest that a man's hairstyle may have gone out of style about the time flagpole-sitting was all the rage. Some men respond to these gentle intimations by redoubling their determination to keep their World War II bomber-ace flattop to the bitter end. Others at first scoff at the suggestion they're behind the times, then privately start to wonder, "Well, could she be right?" How do you *know* if your hairstyle is in style?

It may help to do some browsing before you seek the services of a professional (if that's what you decide to do). Look through men's fashion magazines like *Gentlemen's Quarterly,* or the haircut books you're likely to find lying around a salon, and try to find pictures of men whose hair is roughly the same color and texture as yours. What have they done? Could you imagine yourself wearing your hair like that? Would it flatter your features? Would it be easy to take care of? Does it convey the image you'd like to project to the world?

You might even browse through old photos of yourself to take a look at your personal style history. Has your hairstyle remained unchanged since the Korean War? Are you wearing your hair today as if you still had as much of it as you did when you were 20? Or have you taken to ill-fated attempts to disguise your bald spots, like combing a long straggly strand straight forward over the top? (It never really works.) Perhaps, on the other hand, you long ago abandoned a style that might still really work for you.

The point is that a hairstyle is not "right" simply because it's in style or "wrong" because it's out. Says Francisco: "The most important thing is not to be contemporary but to come up with a hairstyle that really fits your features, that's really flattering to *your* looks."

Sure, looking good is a long way from being the most important thing in life. But if it makes you feel good and contributes to the quality of your life a little, why not do your best to look your best?

MALE PATTERN BALDNESS: IS IT FOREVER?

Oliver Wendell Holmes once suggested a surefire recipe for long life: "Advertise for a couple of parents, both belonging to long-lived families, some years before birth." The same sort of useless advice applies to men who wish to retain a fine, full head of hair to the end of their days: The determining factor in whether you will or you won't is all in your genes.

The gene for "male pattern baldness" (MPB) may come from your mother's or your father's side of the family. But what actually causes this inborn trait to become visible in the form of a receding hairline or a "skullcap" of bald pate is the presence of circulating androgens, or male sex hormones, in your bloodstream. With MPB, healthy hair follicles commit chemical suicide by converting one of these usually harmless hormones into something more powerful—the androgen dihydrotestosterone (DHT). This newly produced substance acts, according to your genetic programming, to shut down hair production.

But what if you're simply unwilling to be satisfied with the genetic fate you were handed? What are the safe alternatives to a hairline that's going . . . going . . . gone?

Over-the-Counter Medications. To put it simply, they don't work. A distinguished panel convened in the late 1970s by the FDA to review all over-the-counter products claiming to grow hair or retard hair loss concluded that none of them did what they claimed (though they were safe for external use). Even

A Cure for Baldness?

Well, not exactly. But the high blood pressure drug minoxidil (sold as Loniten by Upjohn) *does* appear to stimulate hair growth in some men (and women). Upjohn has undertaken a clinical trial of the drug involving 2,200 volunteers, who apply it topically twice daily to their scalps. Early results are intriguing. "I'm not saying we have the answer to baldness yet," one researcher reports, "but in some patients we have grown cosmetically acceptable hair."

Styling Tips for Thinning Hair

- To give thinning hair more fullness, texture and body, apply some styling mousse while your hair is still wet, then blow-dry, being careful not to "bake" your hair by overdoing it, says Pierre Michel's Michel Obadia. Just use your fingers, not a brush, or your hair will end up looking "too perfect," he says.
- "Blow-styling lotions," which come in a pump-operated spray bottle, also add body to thinning hair, says Vidal Sassoon's Francisco. Towel-dry your hair after a bath or shower, mist it with blow-styling lotion, then shape it as you use the blow dryer. These products are water based rather than alcohol based (like hair sprays), so they won't be as drying to your hair.
- Thin, fine hair will look better if you use a styling mousse rather than a gel, because gels tend to plaster down your hair and make it look greasy.
- Many men have the most pronounced hair loss on top of their heads. For that reason a body wave or partial permanent for the thinning hair there may help add body to your whole "look."
- *Don't* let the sides grow long if you're losing hair on top—it only looks scraggly and clownish. Keep the sides short to balance what you've got on top.

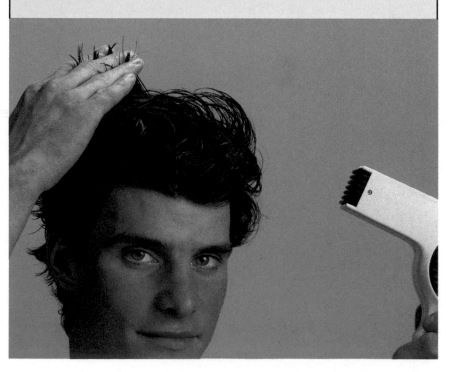

though the FDA announced its intention to remove these products from the market several years ago, the wheels of government turn slowly and it's still possible to buy mail-order potions that may fertilize your geraniums but won't do a thing for your hair. Says an FDA spokesperson,: "The bottom line is, 'Let the buyer beware.'"

Fiber Implantation. Basically, this means implanting hundreds or thousands of colored synthetic fibers directly into the scalp and anchoring them with a knot. It's a resoundingly bad idea. It can cause infection, facial swelling, scarring and permanent hair loss. And on top of all that, most of the fibers fall out as early as two weeks after insertion, often leaving the knots inextricably buried beneath the skin. The cost, by the way, can run into the thousands. "The complications, high monetary cost and ultimate futility of fiber implantation make it an unacceptable procedure," concluded a pair of Cleveland dermatologists after examining 20 victims of local implant clinics. The same procedure using real, individual human hairs seems to produce similar grisly results. One basic problem: "There is no known scientific evidence indicating that hair implants work or why they should work," says an article in the *Journal of the American Medical Association.*

Scalp Flap Surgery. In this operation, a flap of hair-bearing scalp (usually from above the ear) is detached and rotated; the same amount of skin is removed from the target bald spot (usually the hairline) and replaced with the flap, which is sutured in place. This is a legitimate if somewhat drastic procedure, practiced by an increasing number of surgeons. There are several variations—including partial as well as total detachment of the flap. All are done in several steps, taking about a week's time. Cost: $5,000 to $10,000. Advantages: Unlike punch graft transplants, the transplanted scalp flap doesn't lose its hair temporarily, so you get an instant, permanent hairline. On the downside, it's a delicate operation and should be performed only by a skilled (read "expensive") surgeon who's well-practiced in the procedure.

Punch Graft Transplants. Rather than redistributing your remaining hair in one fell swoop, punch grafts do it bit by bit in a series of operations often stretched over 12 to 16 months. Using an instrument rather like a refined cookie cutter, the surgeon takes a tiny circular "punch" of hair-bearing scalp and transplants it where a punch of bald scalp has been removed. This procedure is repeated hundreds of times (typically, 50 to 80 grafts are transplanted in a session). The transplanted hairs fall out in a month or so, and new hair grows in about three months. Though the technique can often produce pleasing results (Senator William Proxmire, Hugh Downs and Frank Sinatra have all had the operation), when badly done it can produce an irregular "doll's hair" look, especially at the hairline, where it becomes necessary to comb the hair forward. The cost per punch graft runs around $20 to $50; since as many as 500 may be needed, the whole production may run $4,000 to $10,000.

Hairpieces. The oldest and still most popular way of disguising baldness is the hairpiece, which has pretty much succeeded the wig. (A wig covers the whole head like a cap; a hairpiece covers only the bald spot.) But since nothing looks worse than an obviously phony head of hair, it's important to get a high-quality hairpiece.

New York's Charles Alfieri, who's been making fine hairpieces for over 20 years, says that the three don'ts are: *Don't* get a hairpiece that's too full—a 55-year-old man walking around with a 25-year-old's hair just doesn't look right (and doesn't fool anybody). *Don't* pick a hair color that's too dark for your skin tone, which tends to lighten as you age. And *don't* get a hairpiece with a hairline that's too low.

Alfieri adds that no really good hairpiece is entirely the same color, since your hair isn't either. At his studio, a hair blender takes samples from the side, front and back of your existing hairline and matches them with the same areas on the hairpiece.

What's the best way to anchor a hairpiece? Alfieri suggests using 3M two-sided nonallergenic surgical tape so that the piece can be easily removed for sleep, swimming or sports. "You see ads that claim you can wear such-and-such a hairpiece while you swim or sleep," he says. "Well, sure they won't come off, but the question is, What will they look like afterward?" A better solution: Get an inexpensive synthetic hairpiece for the gym and save your good one for times you need to look your best.

It *is* possible to more-or-less permanently anchor the hairpiece to your scalp, but doctors take a pretty dim view of this. One method, called hair weaving, holds the piece in place by tying it to your hair. It feels cooler than a taped-on hairpiece, but you can't clean your scalp, and it may encourage further hair loss by pulling on what you've got. Other methods, in which the piece is surgically sutured to your scalp, are even worse because of scarring and the risk of infection.

But even if your hairpiece looks so good only your hairdresser knows for sure—Burt Reynolds, William Shatner and Ricardo Montalban all take their hair off at night—it may still have its disadvantages. Hairpieces tend to be hot and uncomfortable in the heat of summer or in a warm room. They require a good deal of maintenance—Alfieri recommends shampooing every two weeks, as well as periodic cleaning and restyling. They don't last forever—they should be replaced every four years or so. They're a constant source of potential embarrassment (how do you gracefully handle the situation when your hairpiece falls off in public?) And they're not cheap: Alfieri's run from $600 to $950.

SHAVING TIPS: TAKING IT ALL OFF

Is there any *right* way to shave—a technique that's soothing to skin *and* soul? In a word, yes. You may have a personal preference as to your shaving cream or your weapon, but the basics of good skin care still apply to how you use them.

A good blade shave should always begin with the cheapest, most effective beard-softener known to man (in fact, it's the *only* one): water. The hotter the water, the quicker your whiskers will soak it up, or hydrate—but because hot water isn't good for your skin, you should make it lukewarm. Usually about 2 minutes of contact with water is needed to fully hydrate the beard. For that reason, it's a good idea to shave after you shower (or even *in* the shower), if that's convenient. In fact, says a trio of doctors in *The Skin Book*, "you can get a perfectly adequate shave by wetting your face in the shower—no soap or shaving cream is necessary."

Be that as it may, lathering up your face with soap or shaving cream is one of the most pleasant parts of the whole affair. The point of these concoctions is to further hydrate the beard, lubricate the skin to ease the razor's glide and raise the hairs so they're easier to slice. You'll find shaving cream works better if you leave it on for 2 minutes or so before shaving. You could brush your teeth while you wait. Also, try smoothing the lather on *against* the grain of hair growth, to raise the whiskers to the razor.

Which is best—old-fashioned mug soaps, brushless creams or the convenient aerosol can? Let your skin be your guide.

Men with dry or soap-sensitive skin should probably use a brushless cream or an aerosol foam, because these products provide the most lubrication and contain almost no soap (which can be drying). Brushless creams, which come in a tube and are applied directly to the face with your fingers, are emulsions of oil in water and won't rob your skin of its natural oils. Since they don't contain much soap, you'll need to wash your face first, however. To further soothe dry skin, use a moisturizer after shaving, rather than an aftershave lotion.

Aerosols are certainly the most convenient but also the most expensive preshave products—75 to 95 percent of what you're paying for is water and propellant. Those propellants can be irritating to men with sensitive skin, and lime- or lemon-scented creams can sometimes cause phototoxic skin reactions when you go out in the sun. As a general rule, men with sensitive skin would do best to stick with products with the fewest ingredients.

Men with oily skin would probably do better using an old-fashioned shaving soap (the kind you work up to a lather with a brush). These products, being mainly fancified soap, will degrease your face better than aerosols or brushless creams. They're also the most economical of all the preshave preparations (you're not paying for the water), along with being the most drying and alkaline.

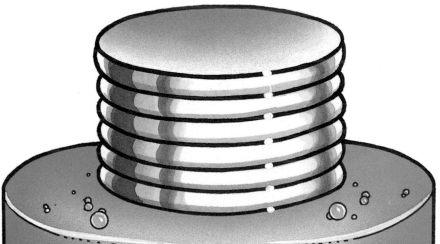

Aftershave Alternatives

It's a zesty ritual most men relish: Slapping a fresh-shaven face with an aftershave. But advertising claims to the contrary, there's no good evidence these products have any particular therapeutic value for your skin. In fact, since most of them are 40 to 50 percent alcohol, they can be very drying (particularly to men with dry skin), and many contain benzocaine (an anesthetic) and other ingredients that can cause painful skin reactions in many people. One alternative is a product like Richardson-Vicks' Saxon Lotion, which has special buffers to prevent or soothe irritated skin, a lowered alcohol percentage (12 percent) and an essential fatty acid, linoleic acid, which heals chapped skin. Or try ordinary witch hazel or Nivea cream, with a few drops of your favorite cologne thrown in.

RAZOR OR SHAVER?

There's no ultimate answer to the question, "Which is best, a safety razor or an electric shaver?" Again, it depends on personal preference and your skin. One study showed that shaving with a safety razor cut hairs cleaner, closer and more uniformly than an electric shaver, which tended to leave the whiskers ragged and split. But then, is the celebrated superclose shave such a good idea?

Men's skin care specialist Mario Badescu claims the search for the perfectly smooth shave is one of men's biggest mistakes, since it can badly irritate the skin and lead to ingrown hairs. Shaving too close "is the main cause of your worst shaving problems," he says. "You're much better off aiming for a mild shave than a superclose one."

Which kind of electric preshave lotion is best for your skin? That depends on your skin. The point of these preparations, unlike the wet preshaves, is to make your whiskers erect and dry and your skin taut and smooth for easy razor glide. You've got two basic choices: alcohol-based lotions or talc-based powders. Men with dry skin should avoid the lotions, advises Dr. Jonathan Zizmor in his book *The Complete Guide to Grooming Products for Men,* because they're more drying than powders. For men with oily or normal skin, he adds, ordinary alcohol "is as fine an electric preshave lotion as any on the market," and much cheaper.

WHAT ABOUT INGROWN HAIRS?

According to current theories about what causes them, men plagued by ingrown hairs on the neck and face are the victims either of genetic bad luck or (more likely) bad shaving habits. Why? Because:

- Shaving *against the grain* of your beard's growth (in practice, this often means shaving upward, especially on the neck) can lead to ingrown hairs since "when you cut against the direction of growth, the hair is cut on a bias or angle, leaving the tip slightly pointed, so it drives back into the skin," says John F. Romano, M.D., clinical instructor in dermatology at New York Hospital-Cornell Medical Center. Learn to shave *with* the grain.
- Shaving *too close* can clip off the whiskers below the surface of the skin, leading to an irritating ingrowth. So shave with a light touch; the less you feel the blade, the better.
- The duller the blade, the more pressure you have to exert, the steeper the angle of the hair's cut edge and the greater the likelihood it will drive back into the skin. Moral: Nothing is more basic to a clean, smooth shave than a sharp blade.
- If you have coarse, curly hair, you'll probably always be more prone to this problem than men with fine, straight hair. One solution: Grow a beard.

STARTING FROM SCRATCH

Many men grow beards just to explore a new look and soon discover that facial hair offers a way of exploring *many* new looks.

But how do you know if a beard is really right for you at all? For better or for worse, you're not the only one who's a party to this decision. It involves whomever you plan to be kissing—and whomever you have to impress. "Beards project an image, and for men in certain occupations, a beard would simply be sending the wrong signals," says Michel Obadia, of Pierre Michel. "Maybe it's not fair, but if you're a banker on Wall Street, people tend not to trust you with $5 million if you've got a beard. Doctors, psychiatrists, artists and creative types can still get away with it."

If a beard *does* fit your lifestyle, how do you go about figuring out what *kind* of beard is best for you? A quick, cheap and painless way to do it is by doodling. Find a photo of yourself (or better yet, several, from several angles), a sheet of clear ace-

Beards have been in and out of style since the time of the ancient Egyptians, who curled, wove and dyed their facial fur into a sort of pendulous braid. Beards were also popular in ancient Greece, where you could tell a man's occupation by the way he wore his beard (philosophers wore them long, historians short). They've been associated with godliness (who could imagine the Almighty without one?) as well as just the opposite (Satan has a neat little goatee). Beards were out of favor during our nation's early days (none of the signers of the Declaration of Independence or the Constitution was bearded). A visitor to Philadelphia in 1794 reported an elephant and two men with beards among the oddities she had seen there.

In recent times facial hair has made something of a comeback, with a Gallup poll reporting that 41 percent of American men now sport a mustache or a beard. No longer a vaguely disreputable symbol of beatnik, Bolshevik or hippie, the beard is just another way of expressing yourself, another way of looking your best, another way of exploring your own style. (And besides, growing a beard is one of the few things left a man can do that a woman can't.) Here are a few considerations to take into account before you decide on a specific style.

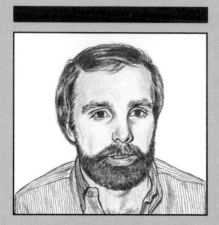

Camouflage

An exaggerated feature like a big nose or protruding ears can be visually deemphasized with a mustache or a beard. The eye will tend to focus on a wide mustache before a large nose or chin. An upper lip that's too thick or too thin can be concealed with a mustache.

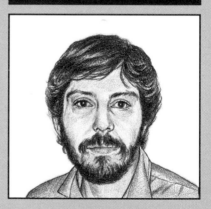

Reshaping

You can "reshape" your face a bit with hairy adornment. A round face can be lengthened with a full, straight beard, or lengthened even more with a pointed beard. A long, angular face can be softened with a rounded beard.

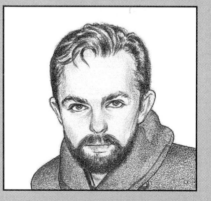

Widening

An overly thin or oval face can be widened with a rounded chin beard worn fairly short and carried all the way back along the jawbone. Anything that gives width to the lower part of the face—even a pair of mut-tonchops—can help.

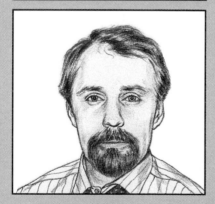

Emphasis

Beards can emphasize a facial feature or hide one. A short, close-cropped beard can dramatically outline but not conceal a strong jawline. A so-called ring beard (a very short beard and mustache that encircle the mouth) can be used to frame a good mouth.

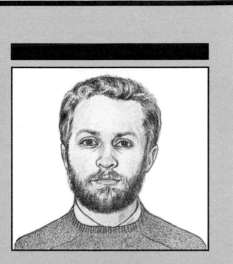

Proportions

A beard must be in proportion to the face and body of its owner. A big man with a round face will only emphasize his size with a tiny Charlie Chaplin mustache. Conversely, a small face or one with undistinguished features will disappear under a massive beard and seem even smaller.

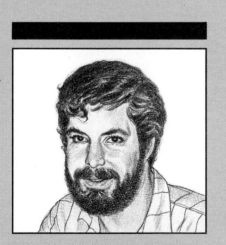

Hairline Match

To some degree, your hairline suggests your beard, since the two of them should harmonize. A low, dark hairline shouldn't be mated with too strong a beard, or it will "close up" your face. A close-cropped beard and mustache can restore visual balance to a face topped by a wide, receding hairline.

tate or plastic, and a black or brown eyebrow pencil, felt-tip pen or china marker. Then set to work like a bored and naughty high-schooler, trying on a bold, drooping field marshal's mustache, then a more conservative one, then a close-cropped jawline beard, a Vandyke, or whatever. Study other men's beards or look in picture books or magazines for ideas.

Naturally, your fantasies will be limited by what will grow on your face: A 23-hair goatee will always look unkempt, so just face it, you can't grow one of those. To find out what you *can* grow, you'll have to live through a few weeks of itchy stubble while the thing thickens enough to sculpt. (To avoid looking like a complete degenerate during the growing-in phase, try getting a fresh haircut and dressing to the teeth.)

When you feel you've got enough hair to work with, wash your face thoroughly with soap and warm water to soften the whiskers. Then rinse, leaving your face wet. Now, use an eyebrow pencil to outline on your face the beard you've envisioned for yourself. Finally, with a sharp razor and a well-lit mirror, shave *away* from the outline with short, careful strokes. And *voilà*—a neatly trimmed beard.

CARE AND FEEDING

Grooming a beard doesn't have to be a big production—just keep it trimmed and clean. The same shampoo you use on your hair normally does fine. "We treat it like any other kind of hair—it's just shorter and slightly rougher than head hair," Obadia says.

For trimming, he prefers to use a barber's comb and scissors for the first "rough cut," finishing up with electric clippers for the finer details. Other men favor the comb-and-scissors approach to the whole job, because by running the comb through the part you want to trim and clipping off the hairs that protrude, you can give yourself a professional trim—and protect against an accidental cut that leaves an embarrassing gouge in your facial finery.

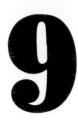

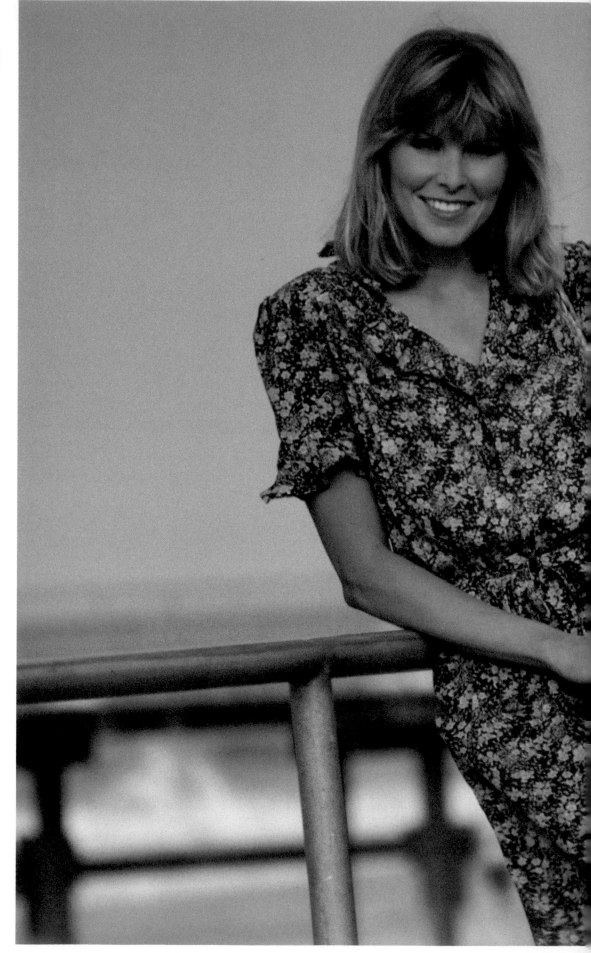

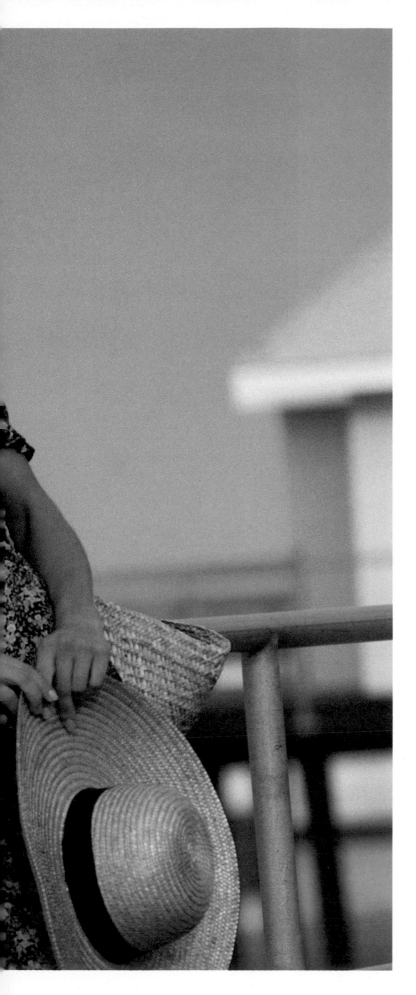

Dressing for Health and Beauty

How to choose clothing and accessories that make you look and feel great, at work or play.

Can you picture Sophia Loren, Greta Garbo or any other symbol of glamour wearing a fur coat and running shoes? Probably not. Yet during the New York City transit strike of 1980, glamorous women of every sort swarmed Manhattan wearing that very ensemble, or one quite similar. Women in other urban areas soon adopted the practical footwear for getting to and from work, and the practice continues today. Suddenly, it seems, perfect taste has taken a back seat to comfort and practicality.

From the simple "survival chic" of a transit strike, a renaissance of practicality has emerged in all facets of dress: Designers and manufacturers began to offer low-heeled dress shoes, topcoats that actually fit over jackets and business suits, hats to warm and adorn and other healthy, rational alternatives to constraining styles, and these alternatives offered new outlets for individuality and flair.

The trend toward clothing that enables you to get around more easily harks back to the dress reform movement of the 1800s, launched by Amelia Bloomer, who invented trousers for women so they could play sports. With the introduction of the bicycle in the 1890s, the freedom of movement allowed by pants made practical, comfortable clothing for women all the more popular. Because clothing that facilitates mobility also allows freer breathing and circulation, it also helped make the wearers healthier.

Intelligently chosen, clothing offers beauty, comfort, utility and durability. Several basic techniques can be used for choosing clothing that works with, not against, your body, beginning with the heating and cooling effects of fabric and clothing design.

How to Feel Neat and Cool When It's Hot and Sticky

Dressing right for hot, humid weather means choosing clothes that work *with* your body's natural cooling system—the evaporation of perspiration—rather than against it. Here are some fashionable hints for staying comfortable.

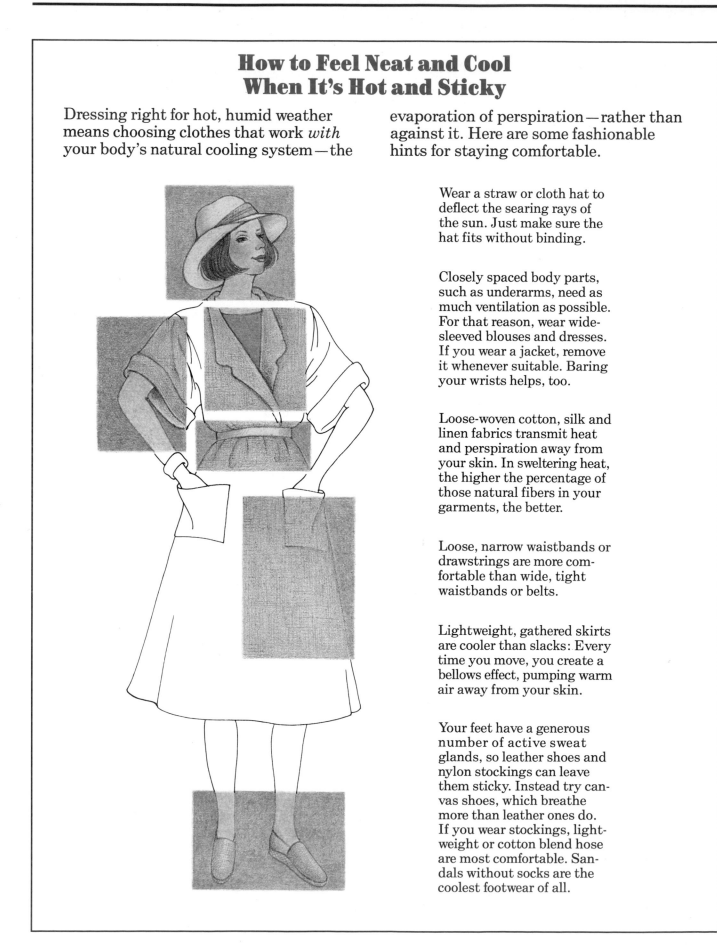

Wear a straw or cloth hat to deflect the searing rays of the sun. Just make sure the hat fits without binding.

Closely spaced body parts, such as underarms, need as much ventilation as possible. For that reason, wear wide-sleeved blouses and dresses. If you wear a jacket, remove it whenever suitable. Baring your wrists helps, too.

Loose-woven cotton, silk and linen fabrics transmit heat and perspiration away from your skin. In sweltering heat, the higher the percentage of those natural fibers in your garments, the better.

Loose, narrow waistbands or drawstrings are more comfortable than wide, tight waistbands or belts.

Lightweight, gathered skirts are cooler than slacks: Every time you move, you create a bellows effect, pumping warm air away from your skin.

Your feet have a generous number of active sweat glands, so leather shoes and nylon stockings can leave them sticky. Instead try canvas shoes, which breathe more than leather ones do. If you wear stockings, lightweight or cotton blend hose are most comfortable. Sandals without socks are the coolest footwear of all.

DRESSING WARMLY, LOOKING LOVELY

Contrary to what you might think, clothing itself isn't what keeps you warm in cold weather. Air trapped within fabric fibers and between fabric and your skin determines how warm you feel. Air absorbs heat from your body, and fabric prevents that heat from escaping.

Some fibers do a more efficient job of keeping you warm than others. Clothing made from plant fibers (such as cotton) and animal fibers (such as wool and fur) are most compatible with your own skin and keep you comfortably warm—for sound scientific reasons. Under a microscope, cotton appears as a rough-surfaced spiral fiber. And wool fleece grows in curly, convoluted locks. When knitted into sweaters or woven into napped or brushed fabrics such as flannel, corduroy or velour, both cotton and wool contain thousands of tiny air spaces that trap and store body heat.

Ever since the last ice age over 250 centuries ago, people living in cold climates also have worn fur. Garments made of rabbit, llama, alpaca and camel's hair and mohair and cashmere (from goats) also work to keep you warm. Like wool, fur traps air.

Synthetic fabrics also have their place in cold-weather clothing. Among them are polyester, nylon, acrylics and modacrylics, all materials made of fibers derived from petroleum. When first introduced several years ago, synthetics brought to mind Dr. Frankenstein's attempt to reconstruct a human: The result was stronger than the original but ill-behaved. Early synthetics did trap air against the skin, but they also trapped moisture, leaving the wearer hot and sticky in summer and cold and clammy in winter.

Newer synthetics such as Orlon, Comfort 12 sweater yarn and polypropylene breathe and allow for the evaporation of moisture, keeping you as warm and dry as natural fibers do. Some space-age fabrics such as fiberfill, Gore-Tex and Damart Thermolactyl perform even *better* than natural fabrics.

Fiber blends, such as polypropylene and cotton, combine the comfort and wicking ability of natural fiber with the strength, durability and easy care of synthetics.

Quilted garments that sandwich fiberfill, down or other voluminous fibers between layers of cotton, wool or nylon efficiently trap great quantities of warm air and are about the warmest clothing you can find.

THE ALL-SEASON WARDROBE

Warm and cold are relative sensations. If the outdoor temperature drops to 60°F on a summer day, you'll feel chilly and grab a sweater. Yet if the temperature soars to 60°F in the middle of winter, you'll marvel at the beautiful weather and peel off your wrap. A wardrobe selected with the vagaries of climate in mind allows you to feel comfortable no matter what the weather.

Layering. Several layers of fabric keep you warmer than one heavy garment because they create more air spaces to hold heat. For example, an oxford-cloth shirt worn over a cotton turtleneck pullover and under a medium-weight sweater will be warmer than a single heavyweight sweater. Layering also gives you the option of shedding a layer or two if the temperature in your office capriciously rises to 82°F in the middle of a wintry afternoon. In summer, a cotton sweater slipped over a lightweight shirt will save the day if the air conditioner is set at a bone-chilling 62°F.

Layering also helps you keep your hands warm without sacrificing dexterity. If you wear mittens over thin or fingerless gloves, you can achieve real warmth—yet a quick yank on the mittens allows you to find your keys or open your wallet without losing *all* your protection.

Loose Fit. Cold-weather clothing should not fit too snugly. A tight fit compresses fibers (especially down and fiberfill), reducing their insulation value. If in doubt over which of two sizes of a garment is correct, choose the larger.

The Inside Story

If you had X-ray vision, you'd see exactly why your feet are happy in low or moderately raised heels—and miserable in stilettos.

4-Inch Heels or Higher

High-rise heels pitch all your weight onto the balls of your feet and your toes, leading to corns and other painful growths.

1- to 2-Inch Heels

Moderately elevated heels distribute weight between the heels and the balls of your feet, taking much of the pressure off your toes. A moderate rise also allows hinged bones within your feet to flex as you walk, improving circulation.

Flat or ¼-Inch Heels

In flat shoes, the burden of support is shifted from the ankles and toes to the balls of your feet and your heels, where it belongs, stabilizing your gait. Your toes are free to help you keep your balance, uninhibited by pain, irritation or swelling.

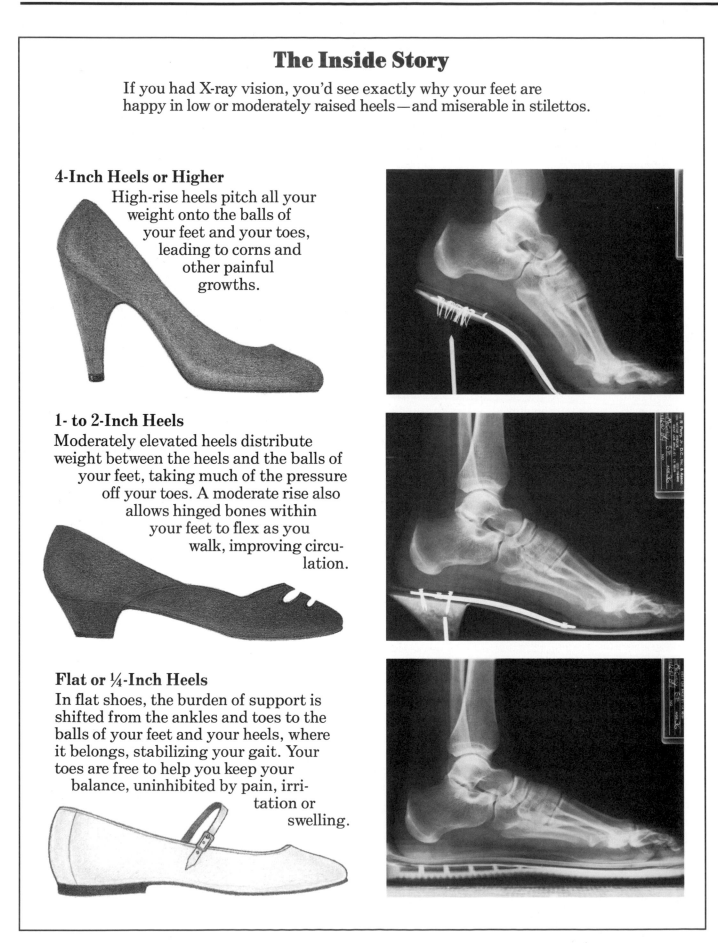

Close the Gaps. Choose clothing designed to seal off points where warm air can escape and cold air can sneak in. Wear scarves or turtlenecks as opposed to open-necked tops, cuffs with knit wristbands or button-down cuff tabs, and jackets with a drawstring or ribbed-knit waistband.

SHOE SENSE

Many shoes look as though they were designed by someone who'd never seen a human foot. Examine the shape of almost any dress shoe. You'll notice that the sole narrows to a streamlined point at the center front. Now examine the shape of a foot. It *widens* toward the front. Talk about trying to fit a square peg in a round hole!

How do your shoes stack up? To find out, try this: Stand on a piece of paper and trace a line around each shoe with a pencil. Then slip off your shoes and trace a line around each foot with a different-colored pencil. If at any point the outline of your feet is larger than the outline of your shoes, you're squeezing some or all of the 26 bones, 56 ligaments and 38 muscles in each foot.

Even worse, this squeeze is exerted under pressure. Take two steps forward, and you bring into play a force greater than your weight on each foot. For example, if you weigh 120 pounds, the ball of your foot may bear about 160 pounds of weight with each step. Take 1,000 steps a day on hard pavement, wearing misshapen shoes, and your feet are bound to hurt. Calluses—patches of tough, dead tissue—build up and may grow inward to form painful corns. Shoes that force your big toes into an unnatural angle may lead to bunions, an inflammation of the joints of your toes and your feet.

Shoes with high heels compound the effects of a tight squeeze. The angle created by the heels pushes the toes forward, pressing against the front of the shoe. The shoe itself is usually made of rigid materials, with thin soles and little to cushion or support your feet. Why does anyone wear these shoes? They're worn because they flatter slender legs by elongating the large muscle running the vertical length of each calf, enhancing natural curvaceousness. Be warned, however, that shoes with very thin high heels and pointed toes exaggerate any extra fullness in the calves, making heavy legs look heavier.

The other lure of high heels is that they temporarily add inches to your height. But the higher the heels, the less stable you are when standing and walking because high heels raise your center of gravity. Standing in high heels, you're forced to lock your knees back, thus straining your ankles and the Achilles tendon in each heel. Any footwear more than 2½ inches high at the heel also forces you to arch your back and stick out your stomach to keep your balance—flattering neither your posture nor your figure.

ANATOMY OF A GOOD SHOE

Most women, of course, will never entirely forgo dressy shoes for sensible oxfords. And you don't have to, because you can minimize the unhealthful effects of high heels by selecting models with elevations of 2 inches or less and following the suggestions given in "Tips for Wearing High Heels." In addition, look for dress shoes with the same qualities that make casual shoes comfortable. Whether you're in the market for pumps, moccasins or walkers, you can find footwear that feels comfortable, wears well and looks attractive if you look for these features.

Ventilation. Uppers made of leather, canvas or other porous materials are comfortable and healthy—they allow heat and perspiration to escape. Uppers made of vinyl, plastic, patent leather or reptile skin, on the other hand, trap warmth and moisture—an ideal climate for the growth of bacteria and fungi.

Cushioning. Cushy crepe and rubber soles absorb some of the shock of hitting the pavement again and again, saving strain on your feet, legs and back. Leather soles absorb some shock, especially if the shoes are lined with foam.

Lightweight running and walking shoes are as close as you can get

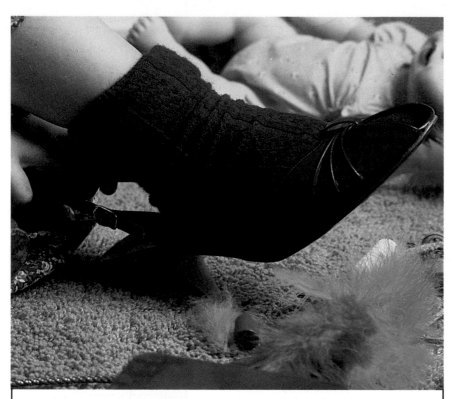

If the Shoe Fits, Wear It

Cinderella's stepsisters weren't the only people ever to have trouble getting stylish footwear to fit. Stores are full of shoes that look awesome but feel awful no matter what size you try. For proper fit, follow this checklist:

- Can you wiggle your toes? There should be a ¼-inch space between your toes and the front of both shoes.
- Does the front of the shoes gently caress your feet, not pinch the sides?
- Are the shanks (the part of the shoes between the ball of your foot and the heel) wide enough to adequately support your feet?
- Does the heel box of each shoe fit snugly, but not *too* tightly?
- Do the shoes feel comfortable when you stand and when you walk, on hard floors as well as on carpet? If not, don't think the shoes need to be broken in. New shoes should feel comfortable right from the start.
- Do the shoes fit well regardless of the designated size? Shoe sizes may vary considerably from one manufacturer to the next, so don't worry if you don't take the same size every time you shop for shoes.

to ideal shoes: As long as they have an outer sole stiff enough to support your bones, soft enough to cushion your joints and flexible enough to allow your foot muscles to flex.

Rigid Shanks. The shank is the area of the shoe between the heel and the sole, located directly under the arch of your foot. Wedgies and other rigid-shank shoes are good because they support your arches. Flexible shank shoes allow the arch to drop, leading to arch strains, heel pain and other problems.

Flexible Soles. Normally, your feet bend like hinges at the ball of your foot. So your shoes, too, should bend like a hinge at that point. Unfortunately, this spot is the widest part of many shoes and therefore often the stiffest.

Side-to-Side Stability. Many shoes— particularly high-heeled shoes—often have convex soles that bow up at the sides, which means that the leg muscles that provide stability have to work continually to stabilize your feet. Not only may your legs become painful and tired, but you're also at risk of spraining your ankles. So look at your feet in a floor-level mirror to be sure the soles of your shoes contact the floor squarely.

What's required for shoes is required for boots, and then some. Located so far from your heart, your feet generally have poorer circulation than other areas of your body (which grows worse with age). Boots, then, shouldn't fit tightly around your calves or ankles. Also, to prevent your feet from becoming damp and overheated, don't wear heavily lined boots indoors all day.

Whether boots or shoes, try not to wear the same footwear two days in a row. Even porous materials need time to dry any moisture absorbed from your feet.

UNDERPINNINGS THAT FIT AND FLATTER

Take any random assembly of women, and chances are that seven out of ten are wearing a bra that doesn't fit correctly, according to International Playtex. One major cause of a misfit is that approximately five out of ten women have an odd-numbered back size measurement (33, 35, 37 and so forth), while most manufacturers make bras only in even-numbered sizes (32, 34, 36 and so on). But there's more to a good fit than odds and evens. To fit you well, a bra should be constructed to fit the architecture of your entire torso. The right bra will wear comfortably and help any bosom, large or small, to look well contoured.

First determine what size bra you should wear—body and cup. Measure the circumference of your torso just below your breasts, at the bottom band of your bra. Add 5 inches to that measurement to get your body size—32, 33, 35 or whatever it may be. If your tape measures an odd number you can ask for a brand made for you, or you can just round up to the nearest even number.

To determine your cup size, measure your bust at the fullest part while you are wearing a bra. The difference between your body measurement and your bust measurement determines your cup size: If your bust is ½ inch larger than your body size, you wear an AA cup; 1 inch larger, an A cup; 2 inches larger, a B cup; 3 inches larger, a C cup; 4 inches larger, a D cup; and 5 inches larger, a DD cup.

Bra cups should completely contain your breast, leaving no gaps or bulges at the tops, sides or breastbone. The back section and straps should not cut into your skin. If the bra rides up in the back, either the bra is too large, the back is hooked too loosely or the straps are adjusted too tightly.

To double-check fit, try the bra underneath a clingy sweater. If the bra fits well, you won't see any extra ripples or bulges, front or back.

Seamless-style bras look smooth and natural under sheer or close-fitting fashions, but seamed bras are made of stiffer fabric and give needed support for a generous bosom. Underwire bras lift the breasts from the bottom and shape from the sides, making the most of a small bust or taking some weight off the shoulder straps for a woman with a full bust.

Nonstretch straps support and stabilize your breasts better than elastic straps, especially if you wear anything larger than a C cup.

"What you want is a bra that allows your breasts and your body to move together," says Christine Haycock, M.D., a trustee of the American College of Sports Medicine.

If you wear a C cup or larger, don't try to squeeze into a smaller bra to minimize your bust. Choose a "minimizer" bra (such as those offered by Playtex), designed to redistribute breast tissue and reduce the bust's projection by an inch or so.

In addition to fit, also consider color. Taupe or other flesh-toned bras are inconspicuous under most clothing—a color that approximates your natural skin tone is less likely to show through white or colored tops. When you wear black or navy blue garments, however, you need to wear a matching bra underneath.

A BRIEF DISCOURSE ON PANTIES AND PANTY HOSE

As with bras, you shouldn't judge panties and panty hose on pretty appearance alone. Fiber and fit are equally important. Above all, be sure to buy cotton briefs or briefs and panty hose with a cotton crotch. Porous fibers allow perspiration to evaporate, whereas nonporous fibers (such as polyester) create a hot, moist environment that encourages vaginal infections. You can minimize the risk of yeast infections in particular if you wear underwear that keeps your vaginal area cool and dry.

If you need support, panties and panty hose with a front panel of Lycra, Spandex or other two-way stretch fiber will help to hold in your tummy.

To fit comfortably and not interfere with blood circulation, briefs should not cut or bind your thighs. And except for bikini-style briefs, the waist should stay in place when you sit, not ride down.

ARE YOU ALLERGIC TO YOUR BAUBLES?

Beads, bracelets, rings and earrings are fun to wear—but not if you

Can Panty Hose Really Energize Your Legs?

Manufacturers of sheer support panty hose claim that their product relieves tired legs. And there's a real physiological basis to that claim. The stockings are partially elastic and tighter at the ankles than at the thighs. So sheer support stockings promote circulation by "milking" your blood upward toward your heart, thereby turning a stroll through a shopping mall into a stimulating massage for your legs.

Support hose help most if you also exercise regularly and elevate your feet periodically. If your legs feel *very* leaden and achy or if you have serious circulatory problems, you probably need firmer support—either thicker panty hose or custom-fitted stockings.

Wear a Hat

Wearing a snazzy hat is a lot like driving a snazzy car: both add flair to your image and perk up your personality. A hat can also keep you warm or cool and protect your hair from sun and drying wind while flattering your appearance.

Hats for Warmth

A busby-style hat of fur or fake fur is about the warmest headwear you can find. A heavily lined beret or fedora of felt, velvet or leather will also do the job, as will a tightly knit, thick wool cap. Be sure the hat you choose covers your head *and* ears.

Hats for Sun

A straw hat with a wide brim or a canvas visor will shield your face from the sun and keep your head cool at the same time. Ventilated baseball-type caps also work, as long as they're made of cotton or other porous fibers, not plastic net and polyester.

Hats for Fun

To find hats that flatter your face and figure, try on different styles at different angles while you stand in front of a full-length mirror. Very wide brims accentuate the bone structure of your face, but tend to make short people look shorter. If you have broad shoulders or a large bust, wear a medium to large hat, in proportion with your upper torso; a small pillbox, for example, would exaggerate upper torso fullness. If you have very delicate facial features, you'll probably look good in a small to medium hat that doesn't overwhelm your face. If the circumference of your head is smaller than average, you may have to ask a milliner to sew an inner band into your hat.

break out in an itchy rash. Sometimes this problem is caused by an allergy to the nickel in your jewelry. (One out of 10 women is allergic to nickel, as is 1 out of 100 men.) Even expensive jewelry may contain nickel. White gold always contains nickel and so does some "pure" gold.

The only way to find out for certain if your jewelry is the culprit is to ask a dermatologist to test it for the presence of nickel. (The test doesn't harm the jewelry.) He or she will dab the jewelry with a cotton swab dipped in a few drops of a chemical called dimethylglyoxime, then add a few drops of ammonia. If the swab turns pink, the jewelry contains nickel.

If your jewelry is indeed the cause of your rash, there's no need to forgo wearing it altogether. Doctors offer the following suggestions.

- Remove your jewelry when you exercise. Sweating and friction promote or intensify reactions to nickel because the chloride in perspiration tends to leach metals from jewelry onto your skin. For similar reasons, don't wear jewelry in a chlorinated pool or salt water; both contain chloride.
- Coat your chains, rings and earring studs or clasps with clear nail polish to create a barrier between your skin and the nickel in jewelry.
- Be sure pin fasteners rest against your slip, not your skin.
- Take your rings off or wear rubber gloves when you immerse your hands in water containing soap or detergent, which can lodge underneath a ring and irritate your skin whether you're allergic to nickel or not. If you wear rings, rinse your hands thoroughly after you wash.
- If all else fails, wear only stainless steel, wooden, copper, plastic or other nickel-free jewelry.

EAR PIERCING MADE SAFE

Ear piercing calls for certain precautions in order to prevent nasty infections and speed healing. Choose nickel-free metals (sometimes termed hypoallergenic) or stainless steel to minimize the risk of an allergic

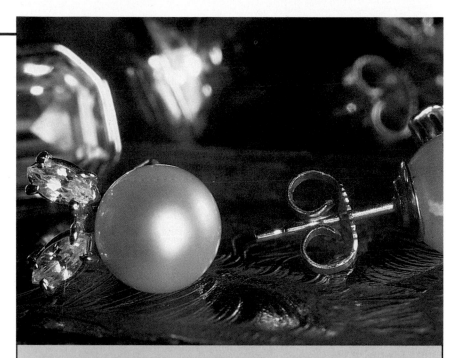

How to Care for Newly Pierced Ears

Freshly pierced earlobes need to be kept clean and free of irritation to avoid redness, swelling and painful bacterial infection.

Insert studs gently, rotating them slightly. Fasten snugly but not tightly—newly created openings need air to heal. Clean your earlobes twice daily: Move the stud first forward then backward, gently dabbing both sides of the opening with a cotton swab dipped in soapy water. Rinse well with a cotton swab dipped in water.

Don't remove your earrings or twirl them during the first 6 weeks, until the openings heal.

reaction. The needle or punch used should also be stainless steel.

Ear piercing is safe as long as the equipment used is sterile. Otherwise, bacteria may enter the openings, making the earlobes red and sore. Untreated, a bacterial infection in an earlobe could spread to the ear itself or to your lymph nodes. So it's safer to have a doctor pierce your ears than to do it yourself or enlist the help of a friend.

If your earlobes feel hard and lumpy, you're probably better off wearing clasp earrings than pierced, because lumps indicate that your sebaceous (oil-producing) glands may have cysts, which could easily become infected if pierced. Also, people who tend to form keloids, or large, unsightly scars, should not pierce their ears.

Shortcuts to Figure-Flattering Styles

Did you ever hear of a diet for broad shoulders? Or an exercise for short legs? Of course not. Some body parts are as unchangeable as your eye color. What's more, some of us will still have bulging tummies or substantial thighs no matter how much weight we lose or how many sit-ups and leg lifts we do.

Clothing can either accentuate or disguise nature's disproportionate arrangements. The wrong styles can make you look broader, shorter or hippier, leaving you with a closet full of expensive mistakes—garments that looked great on the hanger but terrible on your body. The right styles can make you look 5 pounds thinner and camouflage ample areas. In addition to cut, clothing with

vertical lines, long diagonals, tapered lines and mitred stripes create the illusion of length and reduce breadth. Also, crisp, smooth fabrics slenderize, while terrycloth, cable knits and fur add bulk. Small patterns and dark colors can make you look smaller while large plaids, florals or bold patterns can enlarge.

To determine which, if any, portions of your figure dominate the others, stand in front of a full-length mirror dressed in a leotard and tights. Concentrate on the overall profile, not details. Then use the examples given here to wade through the racks of clothing in stores to pick out clothes that work with your figure, not against it—before you even try anything on!

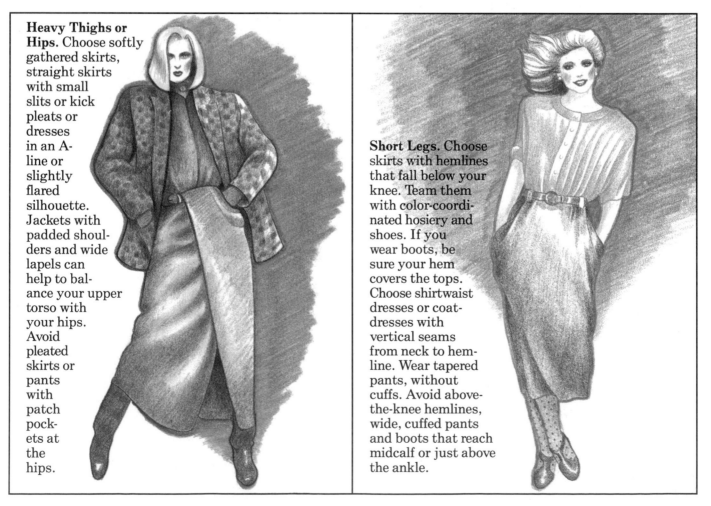

Heavy Thighs or Hips. Choose softly gathered skirts, straight skirts with small slits or kick pleats or dresses in an A-line or slightly flared silhouette. Jackets with padded shoulders and wide lapels can help to balance your upper torso with your hips. Avoid pleated skirts or pants with patch pockets at the hips.

Short Legs. Choose skirts with hemlines that fall below your knee. Team them with color-coordinated hosiery and shoes. If you wear boots, be sure your hem covers the tops. Choose shirtwaist dresses or coatdresses with vertical seams from neck to hemline. Wear tapered pants, without cuffs. Avoid above-the-knee hemlines, wide, cuffed pants and boots that reach midcalf or just above the ankle.

Small Bust. Details such as gathers, tucks, ruffles or shirring amplify a small bust. So do boleros, cable knit sweaters and cardigans, notched jacket lapels, empire waistlines and wide, cinched belts. In short, anything a large-busted person can't wear, you can. Avoid clingy garments that leave nothing to the imagination.

Ample Abdomen. If you bulge below the waist, choose pants in woven fabrics such as poplin, gabardine or wool flannel that hang straight from a tailored waistband. Avoid clingy jersey or polyester knits and elasticized waistbands, which accentuate bulges. Avoid clingy sheaths, belted dresses and dresses with fitted midriffs. Wear control-top panty hose for additional support.

Large Bust or Broad Shoulders. Look for dolman sleeves, blouson sweaters, small collars, vertical necklines, narrow lapels and wrap fronts in straight-hanging (not clingy) fabrics. Avoid wide necklines, puffed sleeves, ruffles, gathers, padded shoulders, wide belts and empire waistlines. Be sure garments don't pull across the bustline or shoulder blades. By all means, wear a good bra with adequate support to minimize drooping.

Short Waist. Overblouses, tunics, empire-waisted dresses and pullovers with dropped waistlines elongate your torso. So does a long scarf worn as an accessory. Avoid belted waistlines, which cut you in half visually and shorten your torso.

Using COLOR to Flatter

Everyone's experienced it. You wear a new sweater one day and friends comment, "You look terrific in that color!"

Let's take that universal experience one step further: Suppose everything in your wardrobe was just the right color. You'd look terrific *every day*.

The women shown here appear wearing colors that are either right or wrong for them. Additional colors that flatter—and light or cool shades of that color—accompany each caption.

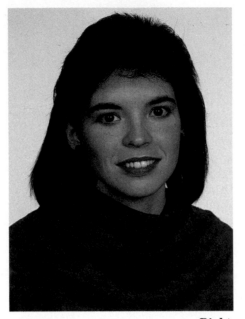

Right

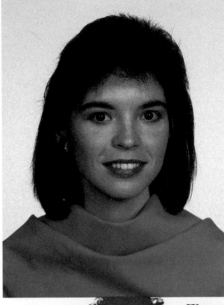

Wrong

Winter

People with cool/dark coloring (also known as "winters") have either dark or milk-white skin (like Jane, above) with blue and red undertones and dark hair with ashen highlights. They look best either in strong colors, such as royal blue (above left), emerald green, red, navy, black or white-white, or cool pastels. Peach (above right), olive and other colors with yellow, orange or brown undertones are less flattering, making the skin appear sallow.

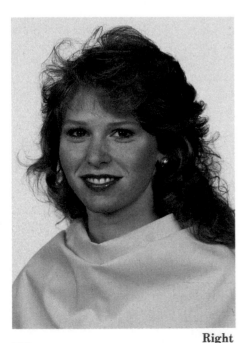

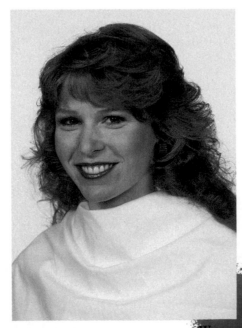

Right

Wrong

Spring

People with warm/light coloring (also known as "springs") have transparent, ivory skin with yellow undertones (like Debby, at left). They look terrific in pale, warm yellow (far left), which plays up warm yellow undertones. So do clear (not muted) turquoises, salmon, camel and ivory. White with no yellow (near left) is too harsh and clashes with Debby's warm yellow tones, so it's not very flattering.

Summer

People with light/cool coloring (also known as "summers") have fair skin with blue undertones and ash-toned hair (like Barbara, at right). They look their best in colors such as bright rose (near right), periwinkle and blue-green, or in pastels such as a cool shade of pink or a soft blue which complement their light/cool skin tones. Green-gold (far right), brown and other colors with yellow, gold or orange undertones clash with blue undertones and aren't nearly as flattering.

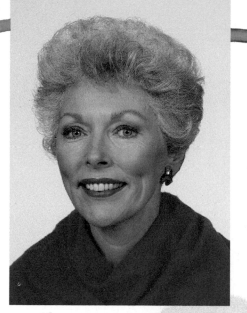

Right   **Wrong**

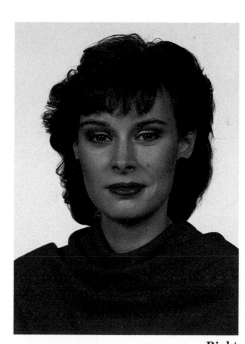

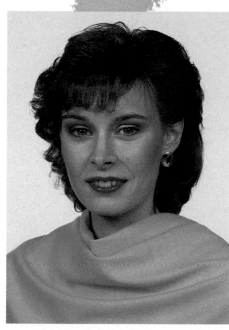

Right   **Wrong**

Autumn

Those with warm/dark coloring (also known as "autumns") have warm-toned skin with yellow-red or gold undertones and gold, red-brown or taupe hair (like Danielle, above). They look great in tomato red (above left) or olive gold, rust, medium to chocolate brown, tan and similar colors that complement the yellow-red or gold undertones. Salmon, coral and peach would also be flattering. Cool colors such as lavender or other colors with blue (above right) or pink are the least flattering.

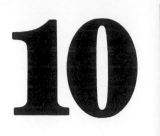

10

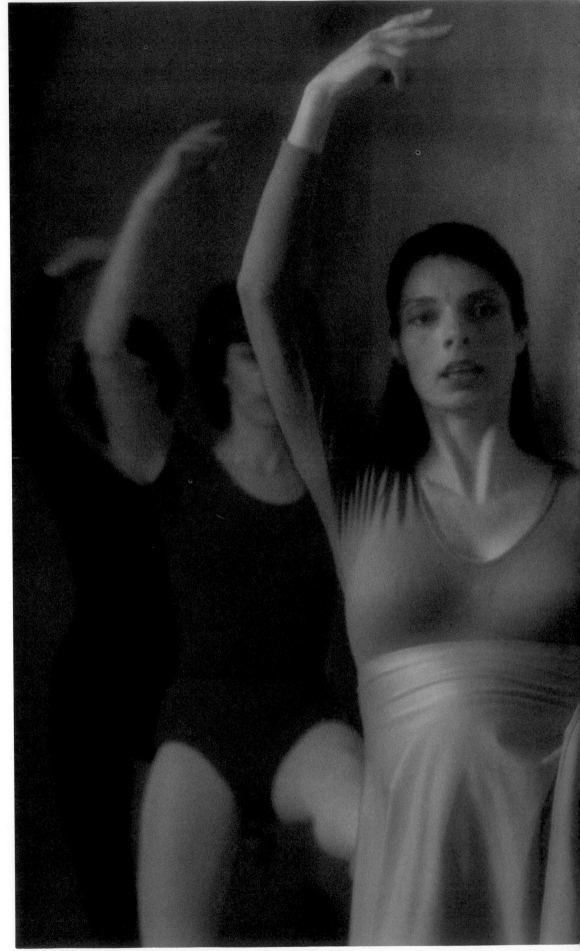

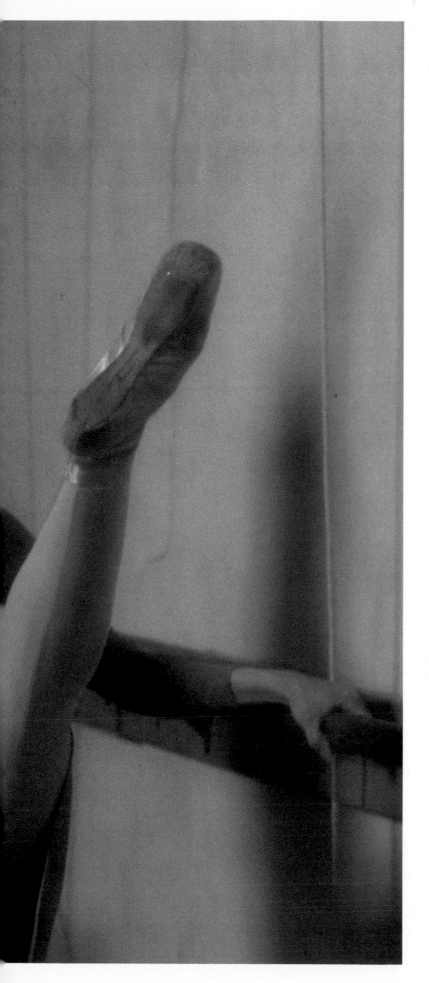

Lady in Waiting

Pregnancy is a special time of feeling and looking wonderful. Go ahead—show off your blossoming beauty.

Despite a rapidly changing shape and some annoying physical discomforts, most expectant mothers fully intend to continue working, traveling, exercising, entertaining and enjoying an active social life. Of course, common sense tells you that certain concessions must be made in order to assure a safe delivery and a healthy baby, but by and large, pregnancy remains a time of staying in life's mainstream and looking one's best: healthy, stylish, even glamorous.

Sometimes, however, the changing hormone levels that jolt your pregnant body can sabotage your best beauty efforts. Your hair may refuse to behave, your complexion may turn blotchy and pimply, or a puffy face and excess facial hair may threaten to send you into hiding. No need to panic. Most of pregnancy's beauty thorns will vanish on their own by the time the baby is six months old. Meantime, some practical tips and cosmetic tricks can help you look your glorious best while awaiting the big event.

TEMPORARY HAIR FALLOUT

One of pregnancy's greatest gifts can be a head of hair that's thick and lush. Whereas normally only from 85 to 90 percent of your hair is in the growing stage at any one time while the other 10 to 15 percent is "at rest" (resting hairs are the ones you find in your hairbrush each morning), pregnancy's hormone surge switches this pattern to nearly 100 percent hair growth. Since hair is largely composed of protein, it is theorized that early in pregnancy, when the tiny fetus doesn't yet have tremendous protein needs, your body can afford to squander precious protein on extravagant hair and nail growth. But this spectacular ratio begins to slide in the second trimester, when the body focuses its energy on a rapidly growing baby instead. Result? From one to five months after delivery you may notice unusual fallout, particularly around the frontal hairline. Happily, the thinning is temporary and self-curing.

Until nature gets back on course, the idea is to get maximum mileage out of thin hair. Now's the time for clever camouflage tactics: Splurge on a professional hair styling and a great cut—or even a hairpiece.

Since thin hair is often lifeless and limp, dermatologist Alan Schliftman, M.D., clinical instructor in medicine at the Albert Einstein College of Medicine, White Plains, New York, suggests frequent shampooing to remove the oil that attracts dirt and gives hair a matted-down look. Follow each washing with a coating of creme rinse, designed to plump up sparse hair and tame the flyaways.

BREAKOUTS AND BLOTCHES

Although nature usually compensates for a ballooning waistline with a complexion that has never looked better, sometimes the reverse is true: Hormonal changes may cause acne and other skin problems to develop.

"Obviously, you can't treat acne in a pregnant woman with many of the medications that might be helpful to someone who is not pregnant," says Dr. Schliftman. (Accutane, for example, may cause birth defects.) Dr. Schliftman also points out that some physicians advise against applying any over-the-counter acne product to blemishes. They suspect that these products may be absorbed by the skin and are, therefore, potentially harmful to the growing baby. "It's best to check with your doctor before using any OTC medication," adds Dr. Schliftman.

Instead, Dr. Schliftman recommends these helpful antiacne measures: Use astringents, which will cause the skin to pull a bit and open up clogged pores. Consult a dermatologist about which moisturizers you can use without aggravating a breakout. Also, substitute water-based cosmetics for the oil-based kind.

As a general rule, pregnancy is a time when everything on the skin tends to grow and darken. Moles and freckles may multiply, scars can enlarge and fleshy growths called "skin tags" may increase in size and number. Often, specific areas of "pregnant skin" take on a darker hue as the result of stepped-up pigment production, according to Sheldon H. Cherry, M.D., assistant clinical professor of obstetrics and gynecology at New York's Mount Sinai Hospital.

Dr. Cherry says that many women first notice signs of this hyperpigmentation on their abdomen, where it's normal for the thin line running vertically from pubic bone to navel—the linea nigra—to darken.

Considerably more public (except to bikini fans), and therefore much more bothersome to a lot of women, is the so-called mask of pregnancy: brownish patches which appear on the forehead, cheeks and nose.

The good news is that there are positive steps you can take to minimize and perhaps even prevent facial skin discolorations. "It's known that sunlight is a major pigment stimulator," says Dr. Schliftman, "and because the skin's sensitivity to sunlight increases with pregnancy, it's best to stay out of the sun altogether or use a sunscreen."

Stretch Marks: Preventable or Permanent?

Stretch marks are so common during pregnancy that many women have come to consider these reddish-purple streaks a "trademark" of the condition.

"They first appear as raised, reddish streaks that can actually be felt if you run your finger across them," says dermatologist Alan Schliftman, M.D., of the Albert Einstein College of Medicine. "Over time, as the inflammation subsides, they will tend to fade. However, stretch marks seldom fade altogether; there is almost always a permanent 'wrinkly' change to the skin."

A genetic component probably accounts for the condition. If the genetic tendency exists, stretch marks probably cannot be prevented, say the skin experts.

If your stretch marks are particularly bothersome during bikini season, you might try a body makeup cover-up cream, especially during the streaky-reddish phase, advises Dr. Schliftman.

If, despite your best prevention efforts, the "mask" appears anyhow, New York makeup artist and skin care specialist Trish McAvoy offers advice on how to make the darkish shadows work *for* you instead of against you. "Most women," she says, "make the mistake of concentrating too much on the problem, which only calls attention to what you're trying to hide."

Instead, start by applying your regular foundation and follow it with just a touch of loose or pressed powder for more opaque coverage. Now, with a suntan- or bronzy-colored blusher, apply, then blend the streaks of color on and around the darkened areas—cheeks, forehead and nose—to give the illusion of a natural-looking tan. It's important to stay with the tone of your problem: suntan-colored blush for freckles and darkened areas, but pink tones for reddish blotches to create an "I've-just-come-in-out-of-the-cold" rosy glow! Save the heavy-duty coverups for very dark patches only.

STAYING FIT AND FLEXIBLE

Being pregnant doesn't alter the need to continue exercising regularly. In fact, according to Dr. Cherry, a certain amount of exercise is mandatory for the mental and physical well-being of a mother-to-be. In addition to preparing your body for the coming challenge of labor, exercise pays off in improved blood circulation, appetite and digestion, as well as more restful sleep.

While skydiving and vigorous horseback riding are obviously to be avoided, most sports—biking, golf, swimming, tennis, even jogging at a mild or moderate pace—are generally permissible. Burton Berson, M.D., director of the Sports Medicine Clinic at Mount Sinai Hospital in New York, cautions against taking up a brand-new sport but says that most activities have the medical go-ahead provided that, first, you were engaged in them prior to becoming pregnant and second, you make any necessary modifications. Dr. Cherry adds that most women who are already accustomed to exercise and sports can

tolerate a more vigorous workout than those who have led a sedentary life, but he emphasizes that walking is an exercise that almost every woman can and should engage in. Working women, in particular, are likely to find that a brisk walk after lunch provides an invigorating and healthful break from their regular office routine.

To be on the safe side, it's always a good idea to discuss your individual exercise goals with your obstetrician.

VARICOSE VEINS

Walking is great therapy for another pregnancy-related problem, varicose veins. Some women are susceptible to developing varicosities in the veins that run down the leg, just under the skin. Heredity and hormones, plus increased fetal pressure on the blood vessels in the pelvic area, can cause blood to back up and the veins to "pop" out. Since the condition is aggravated by sitting or standing in one position for too long, exercises such as walking, swimming, cycling—anything that gets your legs moving—can work to keep blood from pooling in your legs.

Additionally, Dr. Cherry advises wearing elastic support stockings, elevating your legs several times throughout the day and staying within your doctor's weight-gain guidelines. Adds Dr. Schliftman: "Avoid constricting knee socks or too-tight boots. And never sit with your knees crossed."

THE BEAUTY PAYOFF

As you can see, the unique beauty problems associated with pregnancy will probably mean that you'll be spending a bit of extra time on your makeup and grooming. But these are certainly minutes well spent: Looking great helps you to feel great—both physically and emotionally. And the healthy glow of well-being is particularly lovely in a woman who is playing the "waiting game."

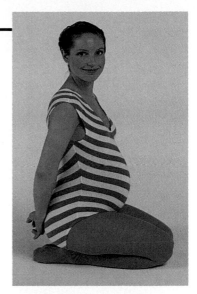

Exercise can help restore your prepregnancy figure as quickly as possible. Walking, swimming and biking help to prevent excessive weight gain and fluid retention during the first few months of pregnancy and to shed unneeded pounds afterward.

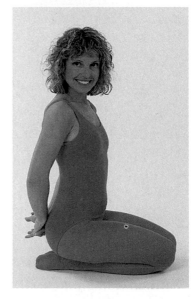

Maternity Wear

Dressing for two is challenging. Coordinating a completely new — yet only temporary — wardrobe requires a game plan.

Above all, maternity clothes should be comfortable. But they also must be appropriate for everything you do: working, playing or going out on the town. What's more, they probably have to take you through three different seasons. That's a tall order.

For help, turn to maternity-wear catalogs. They allow you to formulate that game plan at home. With your feet propped up, you can locate hard-to-find items such as classic suits for women who work.

In addition to new purchases, keep in mind that you can coordinate maternity jumpers, dresses and pants with blazers and cardigan sweaters you already own. In the final months of your pregnancy, perk up your wardrobe with different shoes, hats, scarves and jewelry. Accessories also focus attention away from your abdomen.

The clothes shown here will help you enjoy your pregnancy in comfort and style.

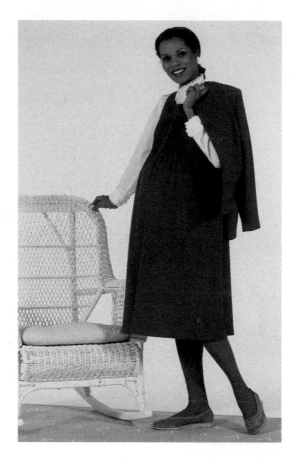

Jumpers are Versatile. They can be worn with a jacket for work, dressed up with a silk blouse for evening wear or dressed down with a tailored shirt for more casual wear. This jumper comes in 7 different fabrics. An adjustable skirt and several styles of jackets are also available in the same fabrics so you can mix and match to form many different outfits. From Mother's Work, P.O. Box 40121, Philadelphia, PA 19106.

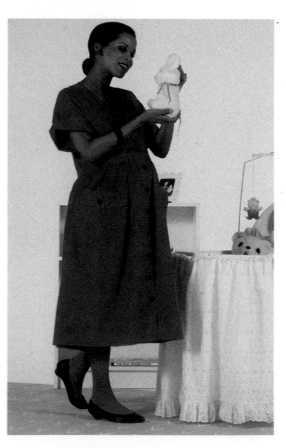

Before-and-After Dress. You won't fit into your normal clothes right after the baby's born, so you'll be thankful for clothes like this flattering maternity dress that doubles as a nursing dress. The front unbuttons to allow you to nurse without undressing. And a matching tie belt adjusts the waistline to fit your changing figure. Available from Fifth Avenue Maternity, P.O. Box 21826, Seattle, WA 98111.

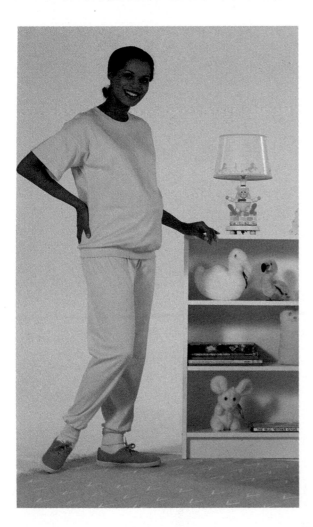

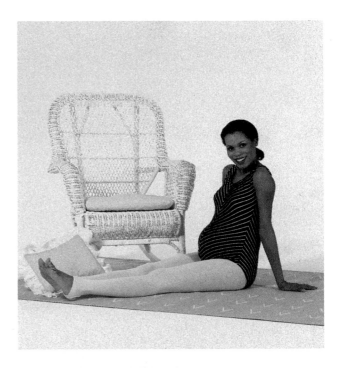

Exercise Clothing. Moderate exercise during pregnancy keeps you looking and feeling your best, but appropriate clothing may be hard to find. Maternity shops now sell leotards and tights designed for exercise during pregnancy, like those shown above. At left is a sweat suit that's so comfortable and spirit-lifting you may want to wear it all the time. It's available from Fifth Avenue Maternity, P.O. Box 21826, Seattle, WA 98111.

Ten-Month Jeans. Even without a stretch panel in front, Levi's Snap-to-Fit maternity jeans will fit right from the first month of pregnancy to the last. They also come in handy after the baby's born while you get back in shape.

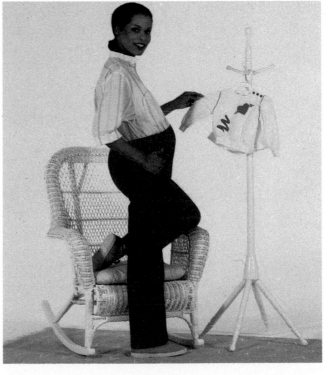

11

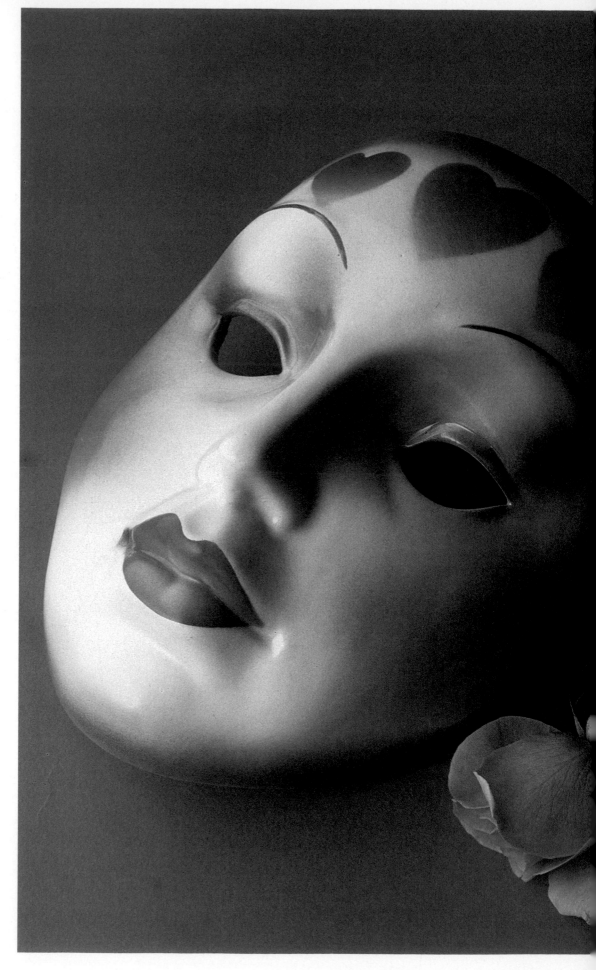

Cosmetic Surgery

This route to beauty is less costly and less risky than ever. But is it right for you?

Who among us hasn't gazed into the mirror and fantasized a new, more beautiful self? Perhaps your imaginary transformation was accomplished with a little lift here, a tiny tuck there, at the hands of a brilliant surgeon. Or perhaps you dreamed of a major overhaul, unsightly ripples of cellulite surgically trimmed off thighs, tummy, rear. For some of us the fantasy is a passing whim; for others it becomes a plan of action.

With modern techniques of plastic surgery becoming ever more refined and affordable, those dreams of a new, more beautiful you seem less remote with each passing year. But accessibility and affordability are only a small part of what you must face if you are giving any serious thought to cosmetic surgery. After all, surgery of any kind is a very serious undertaking, fraught with enormous risks, both physical and psychological. Any potential candidate for a surgical overhaul must weigh carefully the risks to physical and mental health against the rather uncertain payoff in appearance.

How can you tell whether your desire for change is realistic? While there's no easy answer, the first step in your assessment is to form a clear idea of what's involved in cosmetic surgery. Here's a basic primer on what operations are available, their risks, their costs and what results you can expect.

Let's begin with a few words of wisdom from some top specialists.

"The best candidate," observes Dennis Cirillo, M.D., a plastic surgeon in New York City and author of *The Complete Book of Cosmetic Facial Surgery,* "is one who's properly motivated, who has a real and defined anatomical problem and has realistic expectations for what can happen."

PUT YOUR LOOKS IN PERSPECTIVE

Changing a body feature is not a magical cure for a romance turned sour or a lost job.

Why They *Really* Did It

Can cosmetic surgery improve your marriage or land you a better job? Probably not, but it can enhance your self-image. In interviews with 50 female facelift patients before and after surgery, plastic surgeon John Goin, M.D., and psychiatrist Marcia Kraft Goin, M.D., of Los Angeles, uncovered patients' hidden motives for undergoing the operation. Many who had *realistic* expectations experienced an increase in self-esteem and confidence after surgery. Those who were *unrealistic* were often disappointed, not so much with the actual results as with the response they received from the world at large.

"The correct motivation for an aesthetic operation," according to surgeon Goin "is an internal one—to make you feel better about yourself." His psychiatrist wife agrees that a facelift won't change your life by causing someone to offer you a terrific job, "but it may give you the confidence to pursue one."

Here are some of the patients' reasons for cosmetic surgery:

Stated Reason	Hidden Reason
To look better.	Your face looking young can help you to be young; society is youth oriented.
My husband is retiring; I don't want to stay home and grow old.	I had hoped my husband would become more potent. He didn't.
To look younger so as to get a better job.	Young people don't like to talk to people who are old. I don't want my problems to show.
I have a responsibility to look nice for others. (A minister.)	I did it for sheer vanity and now I feel like an ass.
I want to regain pride in my appearance.	I didn't tell you before. I did it to help me get a new job.

How can you tell if you're not a sound candidate for cosmetic surgery? According to Marcia Kraft Goin, M.D., a clinical professor of psychiatry at the University of Southern California Medical School, someone who's in the middle of a life crisis or is depressed or someone who suddenly becomes dissatisfied with a body part that was never bothersome before should carefully examine their motivations. "If you're hoping to save your marriage or escape from feelings of grief or think you're going to get a job by having some sort of plastic surgery, you're bound to be disappointed," says Dr. Goin. If you're feeling depressed, ask yourself: "Am I hoping to solve my depression by having an operation?" If the answer is yes, instead of having surgery, find out why you're depressed and then decide if you want the operation.

Aside from depression, Dr. Goin supports numerous emotional reasons for having surgery. Should a grieving person want an operation as part of the process of getting on with living, Dr. Goin is all for it. Wanting to get rid of self-consciousness, or simply wanting to please yourself (never to placate a lover or a parent), are good reasons, too, she says. Patients who are most satisfied with results are those who are "not looking to solve life's problems by having an operation," says Dr. Goin.

FINDING THE BEST SURGEON

Once you've carefully examined what you expect surgery to accomplish, the next step is to choose the doctor who will work on you. It's essential to find a qualified surgeon who's experienced in the cosmetic procedure you want and in whom you have total confidence.

"First and foremost," suggests the American Society of Plastic and Reconstructive Surgeons (ASPRS), "consult your family physician," or "ask any other physician whom you know and trust," one who is familiar with the work and credentials of several specialists.

If you don't have a personal doctor, you may want to use the referral service offered by ASPRS. Write or call them about the procedure you want done. They'll provide names of qualified plastic surgeons in your locale. (The American Society of Plastic and Reconstructive Surgeons, Inc., Patient Referral Service, 233 North Michigan Avenue, Suite 1900, Chicago, IL 60601; 312-856-1834.) Local medical schools, county medical societies or community hospitals can also provide referrals.

Even better, ask a friend who has had first-hand experience with a plastic surgeon. Dr. Cirillo believes this is the best way to get to the right doctor. "You get to learn not only what the doctor's work is like, but also what the doctor is like," he notes.

In any case, check credentials. Make sure a surgeon is affiliated with a qualified hospital and that he or she is board-certified to do plastic surgery. It's also important to select a surgeon who frequently performs the kind of operation you're seeking.

The final step in making a selection should be based on your personal rapport with your surgeon. Discuss your desires honestly. You should have utmost trust in your doctor's ability to understand and execute what you want. Stephen Genender, M.D., asserts "the difference between a very happy and a very unhappy patient is simply a matter of communication between the doctor and the patient."

A GUIDE TO OPERATIONS

Breast Augmentation (Augmentation Mammoplasty). This is the most frequently sought cosmetic operation. Augmentation mammoplasty increases the size of the breasts or balances unevenness. Usually performed under general anesthesia, augmentation is commonly accomplished by making an incision underneath the breast to create a pocket. A silicone gel prosthesis is then inserted into the pocket and the incision is closed. Afterward, a gauze dressing is applied.

The process takes about 1 to 2 hours and costs $2,000 to $3,000 or more, depending on the complexity of the operation. In many cases, patients can go home the same day.

Within a week, the sutures are removed. Within two weeks, the patient is massaging her breasts to keep the development of fibrous scar tissue to a minimum. Reuven Snyderman, M.D., head of plastic and reconstructive surgery and professor of surgery at the University of Medicine and Dentistry of New Jersey, Rutgers Medical School, points out that "any time you put a foreign substance into the body, fibrous scar tissue will build up around it. Massage helps minimize the problem but occasionally breasts will get firmer than desired and a second operation may be needed."

Eyelid Surgery (Blepharoplasty). This second most common type of plastic surgery is performed to remove excess folds of skin drooping over the eyes, as well as pouches of loose skin under the eyes. Often it's done in conjunction with a facelift. The procedure costs about $2,000 to $3,000, can be done under local anesthesia and normally takes about 1 to 2 hours. Recovery takes about two weeks and the hairline scars fade within a couple of months.

Facelift (Rhytidectomy). The classic lift is done by separating the facial

Smoking and Facelifts

"Smoking can be hazardous to your facelift," concludes Thomas D. Rees, M.D., a plastic surgeon affiliated with the Manhattan Eye, Ear and Throat Hospital. In a review of the records of 1,186 patients who had a facelift, Dr. Rees confirmed a direct association between cigarette smoking and the ability to heal following the surgery.

Among the records reviewed, Dr. Rees found 121 patients who had evidence of skin slough, the shedding of dead tissue caused when a significant portion of blood supply fails to reach the skin. The result is delayed healing and more noticeable surgical scars. Dr. Rees contacted 91 of the patients on record, 73 of whom admitted to smoking more than a pack of cigarettes a day.

Alternatives to Surgery

You can improve your appearance in a variety of ways that are less drastic than surgery. Here are some options to consider.

Chemical Face Peeling

According to Barry Martin Weintraub, M.D., a plastic surgeon based in Beverly Hills and Manhattan, chemical face peeling is best for fine facial wrinkles, superficial acne scars, blotchy skin or the discoloration often seen under the eyes. The process uses a chemical preparation to create a burnlike reaction on the upper layers of the skin. When these layers peel, the new skin that grows back has a smoother, finer, rejuvenated look.

Dermabrasion

This procedure is best for the removal of acne pock marks, wrinkles of varying depth and superficial tattoos. The surgeon uses a dermabrader, a high-speed electrical device that removes the upper layers of the skin with brushes, wheels and sanders. This technique also causes the skin to peel, revealing smooth new pink skin beneath.

Lasers

Lasers remove skin discolorations such as port-wine stains from birthmarks. Some people believe that the laser-beam technique can be used to provide a "nonsurgical" facelift by directing the laser at acupuncture points on the face. However, some plastic surgeons assert that lasers directed toward these points do not result in a "lift," and warn against such erroneous claims.

Collagen Injections

According to Dr. Weintraub, collagen injections are the safest, easiest, most dramatic way of getting rid of wrinkles. Collagen augments the fabric of your skin, thereby filling in wrinkles. It is a natural protein, purified and stabilized from calf hide and easily integrated into the human skin. When done properly by an expert, collagen injections are safe. The treatment is not permanent, however, and touch-ups may be necessary after only 6 months.

skin from the muscle beneath and pulling the skin tight. Incisions are made along the sides of the face, hidden inside the hairline. The procedure can be performed under general or local anesthesia.

A slightly more extensive—and more long lasting—procedure involves removing accumulations of fat from the neck and jowls and tightening connective tissues and muscles. The cost can run from $3,000 to more than $5,000, depending on the extent of the operation, which can take from 2 to more than 4 hours.

Swelling, skin discoloration and some pain are common after surgery. Dressings are usually removed in a few days. If hospitalization has been recommended—facelifts also can be performed in a surgeon's office or in a surgical facility—you'll be released in two to four days. Recovery takes about three weeks.

Surgery for the Nose (Rhinoplasty). It's performed under local or general anesthesia and costs between $1,500 and $3,000. Incisions are inconspicuously made inside the nostrils; cartilage and bone is cut and chiseled to form the desired appearance. Outside incisions are made only if flared nostrils are being narrowed.

For the first few weeks after surgery, physical activity is restricted. Swelling and bruising will subside within a few weeks. However, healing is gradual and the final result may not be fully discernible for weeks or even months after the operation.

Body Contouring (Suction Lipectomy). Unwanted "love handles," a bulging abdomen, fatty deposits on thighs, buttocks or arms can be eliminated through suction lipectomy ($1,000 to $3,000 or more, depending on the extent of the surgery). The surgeon first separates the fat to be removed by making small incisions and then passes a tubular instrument into the tissue under the skin. Within about an hour or two, the fat is "vacuumed" away via a suction process.

WEIGH THE RISKS

No surgical procedure is free of risks, and cosmetic surgery has its share. The most basic problems that arise in any form of surgery can range from complications due to anesthesia to hematomas (localized collections of blood) or delayed healing, which can cause excessive scarring. In addition, each procedure carries risks of its own. In facelifts, for instance, you can suffer permanent nerve damage, blood clots, hemorrhaging or sloughing of the skin, which creates scars. With breast augmentation, risks include infections, hematomas and loss of sensitivity in the nipples.

Fortunately, most complications are rare in the hands of qualified surgeons, but they can happen and you should be aware of them.

To avoid one type of complication, Dr. Snyderman strongly recommends donating your own blood for surgery (autotransfusions) to ensure a supply when you need it and to reduce risk of contracting disease. You'll need to donate blood two weeks and one week before surgery. Then, on the big day, you'll enter the operating room with two units of your own blood available. Dr. Snyderman feels this offers the patient an added benefit, since a surgeon will be more inclined to use blood if it is the patient's own. "We find the patient whose blood level is kept up by replacing blood lost during surgery recovers quickly, is up and walking around the next day, and generally feels better," says Dr. Snyderman.

HOW MUCH WILL IT COST?

Prices vary according to procedures, surgeons and location. In addition to surgical fees, you'll pay for anesthesia and hospitalization (if required). Payment is almost always requested in advance.

Insurance plans rarely cover cosmetic procedures done solely to improve your appearance. (However, medical expenses can be deducted on your income tax.) Reconstructive surgery often is covered. In recent years the distinction between cosmetic surgery and reconstructive procedures has been blurring. Some surgical procedures previously thought of as aesthetic are now considered reconstructive and are covered by insurance policies. For instance, if a woman has limited physical activity and discomfort from breasts that are too large, reduction mammoplasty may be a necessity, and therefore eligible for insurance coverage.

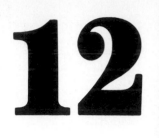

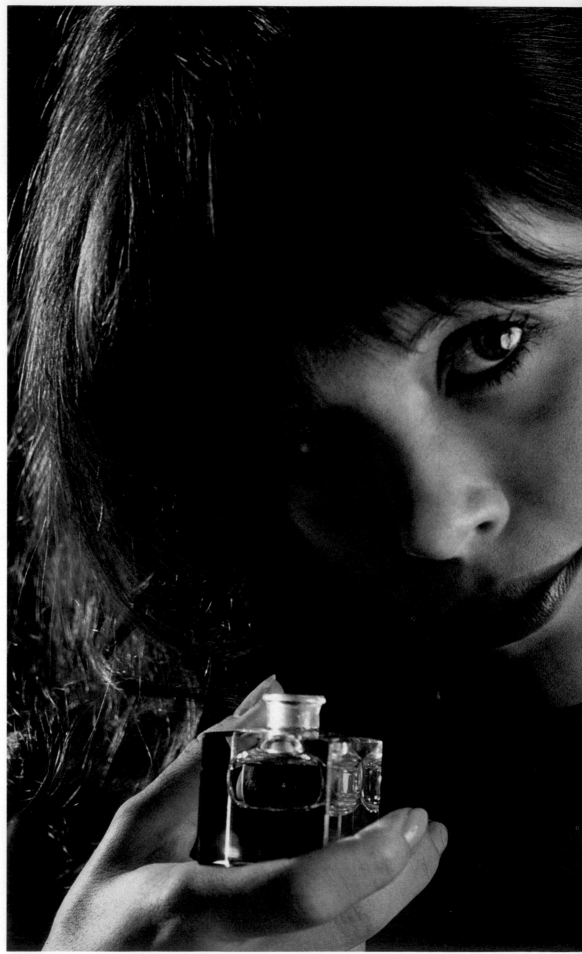

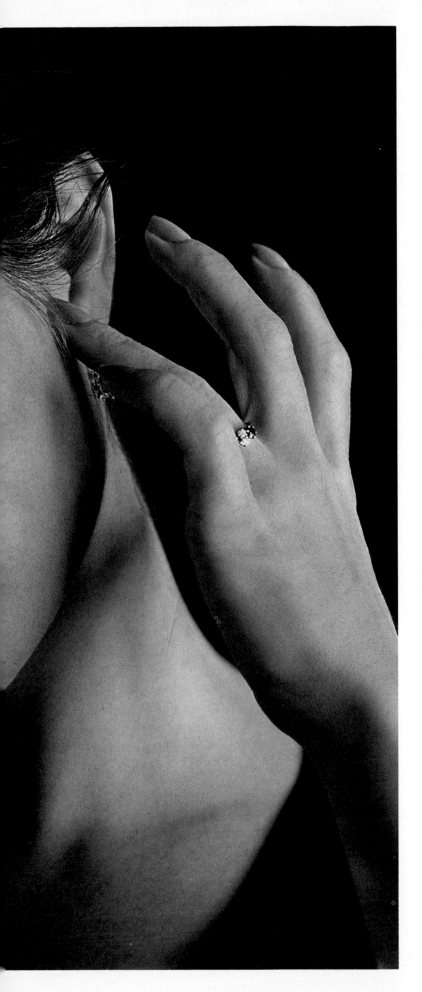

Finishing Touches

If you're well groomed down to the last detail, you'll look good in either jeans or an evening dress.

Word has it that Cleopatra scented the sails of her barge to command attention as she arrived in various ports. On a less grandiose scale, a drop or two of pungent, long-lasting perfume dabbed behind your ears can create a special aura in the air around you. Wearing a fragrance is one of several finishing touches that marks you as an individual.

Other subtle touches also contribute to overall beauty in small but significant ways. Think about the way you sound: If your voice is charming and pleasant, others will be inclined to listen to what you have to say. A neat manicure gives the impression that you take pride in details, be they personal or business. Eyeglasses, too, are as integral to your appearance as your makeup or hairstyle. With the right frames glasses can *flatter* your face, not detract from it.

Details. Put them all together, and details like those work together to make the difference between looking good and looking *terrific*.

Once you develop the habit of taking care of details, those finishing touches simply become part of your routine. Regular manicures and other grooming procedures won't necessarily take inordinate amounts of your time. For example, buffing your nails lightly and pushing back the cuticles, plus a few minutes of proper filing, may be all you need to keep your nails fit and trim.

Don't worry about being considered vain for spending a little extra time on finishing touches. Quite the contrary. Attention to detail is often viewed as the mark of an organized individual who not only has self-respect but usually respects others as well. And, like makeup and hairstyling, many of these good grooming practices also can affect your health.

THE MAGIC OF SCENTS

Scents add to your sensory image: Your choice of fragrance can declare your mood or personality. If

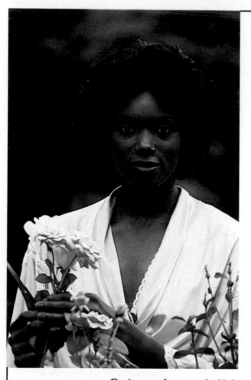

How to Choose a Scent That's Right for *You*

Whether you always wear your own special "signature" scent or match different fragrances to your moods, knowing the basic personalities of scents helps you to choose. *Single florals* are simple scents derived from the essence of a single type of flower —roses or gardenias, for example. *Floral bouquets* are harmonious blends of floral essences. *Orientals* are full-bodied, exotic fragrances often containing musk or amber. *Spicy scents* are derived from cinnamon, cloves, ginger or other spices and sometimes from spicy-smelling flowers. *Woodsy-mossy or forest scents* are earthy, outdoorsy aromas of ferns, sandalwood, balsam and oakmoss, among others. *Fruity blends* capture the fresh, warm scents of citrus or peaches. *Modern blends* are slightly more complex fragrances—often based on traditional scents but each developed to have its own singular aroma.

You can't judge a scent's true character by sniffing fragrance from a bottle. Dab a little on the inside of your wrist for a better idea of how the fragrance will smell on *your* skin. And don't sample more than 3 scents at one time—you'll confuse your sense of smell.

you're feeling sweet you may want to wrap yourself in floral scent. A sultry mood might be signaled by an Oriental blend. And a crisp, clean, woodsy smell can be just right when you're in the mood for the great outdoors. Regardless of which fragrances you choose, it's important to know the difference among various types of scent and something about the way they behave—and vary from person to person. Understanding the nature of the product can help you wear scents to your best advantage.

A *perfume* is a rich blend of natural oils, synthetic chemicals diluted in alcohol, and substances known as fixatives to help the scent last once it's applied to your skin. Perfumes are heavy, best worn in the evening or in cool weather. *Colognes* are comparatively light, subtle blends of oils and alcohol—diluted perfume, really—that are perfect for daytime or warm weather.

Whatever type of scent you choose, part of its beauty is that it develops a slightly different aroma or intensity with each person who wears it, as the oils mingle with skin oil and interact with individual body chemistry. As a matter of fact, fragrance lasts longer on normal or oily skin than on dry skin.

Apply fragrance to your pulse points—behind your ears, at your temples, on your wrists, at the base of your throat and over your heart. Warm spots allow scent to develop fully. And remember this general rule: A little goes a long way.

To prevent changes in aroma, keep your perfume or cologne out of direct sunlight and away from heat. If your perfume has a stopper, wipe it clean every so often to prevent residue buildup that could change the aroma.

DOS AND DON'TS FOR STRONGER, PRETTIER NAILS

Having great-looking nails depends on more than a few strokes of dazzling color. Your nails, like your skin and hair, need careful grooming to look and behave their best.

Your nails consist of hardened protein cells called keratin. Substances called fatty acids keep nails flexible, so they don't break each time you type or dial the phone. Surrounding each nail is the cuticle, which protects your nail bed from infection.

Detergents, chemicals and solvents (even solvents sometimes found in nail care products!) can weaken nails. So can prolonged or frequent exposure to water. If nails split at the least provocation or just don't seem to grow, they may simply need *protective* grooming habits. To help your nails look their best, heed these dos and don'ts.

Dos:

- Wear protective gloves for house-work or whenever your hands are in water.
- Insert your fingertips in half a lemon and twist your fingers back and forth to clean your cuticles and nails before a manicure.
- File your nails into squarish ovals, not points. Slightly squared corners absorb impact more evenly than points, preventing splits and breaks.
- Choose pale or neutral shades of polish. Slight nicks will be barely noticeable and quick touchups will be easier than if you wear dark shades of polish. These touchups not only prolong the life of your manicure, they also prolong the life of your nails. They cut down on the frequency of contact with polish remover, which, if used frequently, can dry your nails and leave them brittle.
- Apply a topcoat (a clear form of polish) over nail enamel to add luster and help prevent chipping.

Don'ts:

- Never peel off nail polish. Along with it, you'll peel off the thin, protective, topmost layer of your nails, weakening them.
- Don't use cuticle remover creams. They usually contain sodium or potassium hydroxide (a form of lye) or other agents that can not only irritate your cuticles but also soften your nails right along with your cuticle. A regular moisturizing lotion will do a fine job of grooming cuticles, with no adverse effect.
- Avoid abrasive buffing creams, which can thin your nails.
- Don't wait for your nails to grow long before wearing polish. A neat manicure, including polish, protects your nails and helps them to grow longer. You're also less apt to bite your nails if you have a nice manicure.

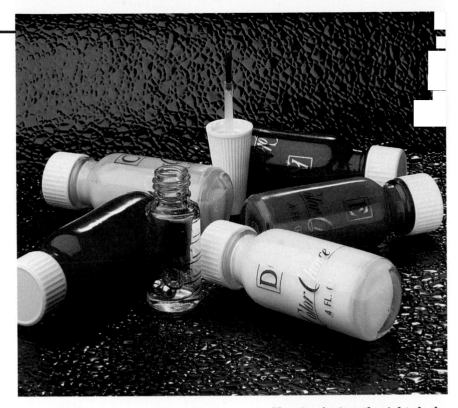

- Don't be tempted to glue fake nails to your fingertips. Plastic nails can loosen easily. (They have been known to fall into the shrimp dip or slip off when shaking hands with a prospective employer.) Aside from the potential embarrassment they may cause, artificial nails can cause other problems—the glue can cause skin inflammation.
- Avoid sculptured nails, too. These are made with several applications of liquid resins that mold to the shape of your own nails and harden. Sculptured nails may split and thin the natural nail and may cause allergic skin reactions. Better to cultivate your own, beautiful nails.

EASY SOLUTIONS FOR PROBLEM NAILS

If you take reasonably good care of your nails and still aren't satisfied with their condition, don't give up hope. Specific problems call for specific added cautions and advice.

Brittle Nails. If you suffer more than an occasional split or broken nail, your nails are probably dry. To help seal in protective fatty acids and slow dehydration, coat your

(continued on page 158)

Five Steps to Perfect Nails

Well-groomed nails make your hands and feet look great. Yet you may not have either the time or money to invest in a professional manicure or pedicure. No matter. With equipment you probably already have on hand, you can—easily, by yourself and at home— make your nails look wonderful.

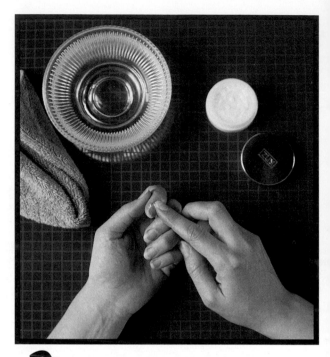

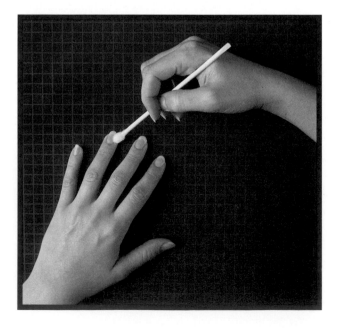

1 Begin your manicure by removing any old nail polish. With an emery board, file your nails at a 45-degree angle in one direction—never back and forth—from the outsides of your nails to the centers. Don't file your nails down to the corners.

2 Soak your fingertips for about 2 minutes in a bowl of lukewarm water and a teaspoon or so of baby shampoo. Scrub them lightly with a soft nail brush. Rinse, then pat your nails dry. Massage hand lotion or cream into the sides and base of each nail.

3

With an orange stick wrapped in cotton gauze, gently push back your cuticles. Never use the pointy end of a nail file or anything that can dent or put ridges in your nails.

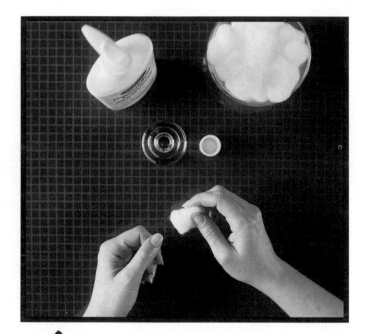

4

With a chamois nail buffer, buff your nails diagonally, in one direction only, using long, even strokes. Be careful: If your nails feel warm, you're buffing too vigorously and generating friction.

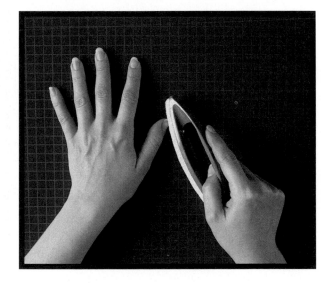

5

Polish does more than adorn your nails; it also helps protect them against detergents and prevents chipping. For further protection against chipping, apply a basecoat, a clear polish that helps enamel to adhere easily. Slick the polish over this base. To discourage split nails, wrap both basecoat and polish around the tip of each nail.

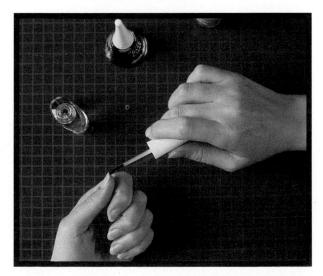

Six Simple Steps to Prettier Feet

Treat your feet to regular pedicures— every 2 weeks or so—and they will be as well groomed as your hands. A pedicure is much like a manicure, with a few added steps.

1. Soak your feet for 5 minutes in a basin of warm, sudsy water that has been enriched with a few drops of baby oil to soften your skin. Rinse your feet and dry them thoroughly, especially between your toes.

2. Smooth away any rough spots on your toes, heels or soles with a pumice stone. (Never cut corns or calluses with a razor blade.)

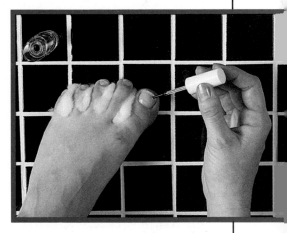

3. Clip your toenails straight across and smooth them with an emery board.

4. To polish your toenails, separate your toes with thick wads of cotton or a foam-rubber toe separator or weave a tissue in and out between the toes.

5. After filing and painting your toenails and allowing them to dry thoroughly, massage your feet thoroughly with a rich moisturizing lotion.

6. Between pedicures, apply lotion after each bath or shower—especially where calluses tend to form—to keep feet smooth and soft.

nails with a commercial nail hardener. If you'd like to experiment with a new approach, soak them in warm water for as long as you can manage (2 hours is ideal) then coat each nail with a drop or so of mineral oil and rub it in well. Also, be sure to file your nails with an emery board—it's gentler for your nails than a metal file.

Pits or Horizontal Ridges. Often, pits or ridges are caused by pushing the cuticle back too hard or using too sharp a manicure tool, which can dig into the nails where they're the softest. Then, as your nails grow out, scars appear as pockmarks or raised ridges. Massage cream on the nails and against the cuticles with a cloth. Push cuticles back very gently with an orange stick wrapped in cotton. Marks should disappear in four or five weeks.

Broken Nails. If one of your nails breaks way below the tip of your finger, you don't need us to tell you it hurts. Besides feeling sore, though, your injured finger also will be prone to infection and further injury should the nail catch on clothing, for example. To protect your finger while your nail is growing back, ask a salon operator for a nail wrap. In this process, what's left of your nail is splinted with a piece of cotton, silk, paper or other fibrous material that is cut to fit and applied to your nail with special glue. Smoothed, shaped and polished to look like your own nails, the wrapped nail will last a couple of weeks longer—long enough for it to grow out.

Wipe Out Perspiration Stains

Both perspiration and the products used to control it can leave stubborn stains or odor in the underarms of garments. To save them from permanent damage, the International Fabricare Institute offers these tips.

Use an antiperspirant. Apply just enough to keep you dry, but no more. And allow the product to dry before you dress.

Use a waterproofing spray on garments. Check the label to be sure which fabrics the spray will safely protect.

Flush out underarm areas of clothing with warm water before washing. Then launder garments in the hottest water appropriate for the fabric, and don't skimp on detergent.

To remove stains in cotton, cotton/polyester blends, nylon, linen or ramie, mix ½ cup of powdered dishwasher detergent in 1 gallon of water. Bring the solution to a boil, remove it from the heat and soak the stained garment for 30 minutes.

Wear dress shields or lightweight cotton T-shirts underneath silk or wool, fabrics particularly susceptible to perspiration damage.

If all else fails, take the stained garment to a dry cleaner and point out the problem. Certain acidic solvents sometimes can remove these stains.

DEODORANTS THAT WON'T LET YOU DOWN

To effectively control underarm wetness and odor, it helps to understand sweat. Did you know, for example, that perspiration itself has no odor? What makes it smell is the bacteria working on it. You probably *do* know that exercise and hot weather prompt your sweat glands (some of which are located in your armpits) to spurt perspiration—tiny geysers of water and salt that cool off your body.

But science tells us that hard work, strong emotions and other forms of stress also force your body's apocrine glands (sweat glands located primarily in your armpits) to release tiny droplets of milky, odorless sweat. Bacteria lounging on the skin surface interact with apocrine secretions, giving off odors variously described by "odorologists" as being as mild as overripe peaches or faintly goatlike, among other terms.

Women have fewer and smaller sweat glands and as a rule, generate less odor and different scents than men do. In fact, studies have shown that when presented with various sweaty T-shirts, some individuals can identify which shirts were worn by men and which by women—attesting to the biological fact that underarm odor served, in part, as a means to identify and attract the opposite sex.

Biology lessons aside, most people want to banish wetness and odor as completely as possible. Hence the overabundance of deodorant and antiperspirant creams, lotions, roll-ons, sprays, powders and sticks on the market.

The ideal underarm product neutralizes odor for hours, dries quickly and invisibly, stops wetness and won't stain clothing. Does such a product exist?

Antiperspirants and combination deodorant/antiperspirants contain aluminum salts, which shrink the openings of your sweat glands to reduce the flow of perspiration for several hours. And they contain antibacterial ingredients to decrease bacteria and control odor. If you perspire excessively, look for an antiperspirant made with a higher concentration of aluminum chloride.

Some deodorants, too, contain antibacterial or antimicrobial ingredients such as triclosan that decrease bacteria and neutralize odor but don't stop perspiration.

Roll-on and cream products protect better than other types because they are water based. By comparison, sticks are alcohol based and dry more quickly than liquid deodorants or antiperspirants. Aerosol products also dry quickly, but some scientists are concerned that aerosols endanger the lungs if you inhale the particles.

"It's a rare person who cannot control odor and wetness with an underarm product of some kind," says James Leyden, M.D., chief of the dermatology clinic at the University of Pennsylvania School of Medicine.

DRYNESS WITHOUT IRRITATION

The U.S. Food and Drug Administration reviews antiperspirants for safety and effectiveness. So you needn't worry that blocking your sweat glands will harm you.

"Antiperspirants inhibit only 30 to 40 percent of total body perspiration, and that's not enough to

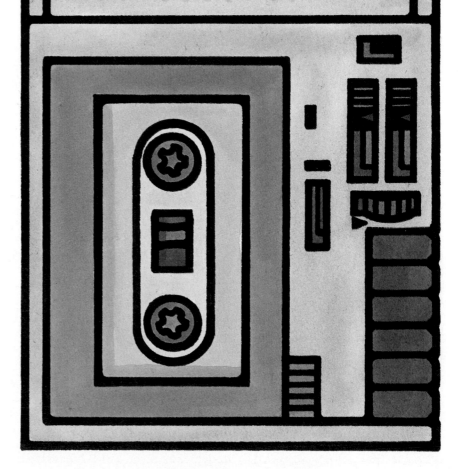

Grooming Your Voice

Your voice is your "second face," almost as important to your appearance as your eyes, lips and skin. Such an important aspect of appearance merits a lot of care. Yet many people don't give their voices any thought at all. Because vibrations within your head prevent you from hearing your voice the way others do, you may not know if your voice is shrill, or if you have unflattering speech habits that may strain or irritate your vocal cords—permanently.

Could your voice use some polish? To find out, tape-record yourself participating in a meeting, engaging in dinner conversation or reading aloud from a newspaper. Listen for the following characteristics.

Volume. A pleasant voice is neither too loud nor too soft.

Pace. Do you speak too quickly? Or slowly and monotonously?

Clarity. Do you pronounce every word clearly?

Pitch. To test the pitch of your voice, say "umm-hmm" to yourself as though you are agreeing with someone. You should feel a slight tingling around your nose and lips. If your throat tingles, the pitch of your voice is too low.

Practice speaking into a tape recorder 10 minutes a day and monitor your voice. Your goal is not to adopt an artificial voice, but to train your natural voice to serve you best.

Choosing Eyewear

Look for the size, thickness and color of frames that suit your complexion and facial structure.

Generally, the distance between the upper and lower rims of your frames should equal approximately one-sixth the length of your face from chin to hairline. Lightweight frames suit slender features. The larger your bone structure, the thicker your frames should be.

The color and shade of your frames should complement your skin and hair color, not match your wardrobe. For example, light brown frames harmonize with fair or ruddy skin and with blond or red hair. Dark brown frames suit warm, dark complexions and brown or black hair. Gray frames flatter those with gray hair and warm tones, while cordovan and other shades of red suit people with gray hair and cool-toned skin. Black frames are somewhat neutral and look good on nearly everyone.

significantly interfere with the body's natural production of perspiration," says Dr. Leyden.

Irritation or rashes from underarm products are not unusual, though. If you have sensitive skin, look for antiperspirants that contain aluminum chlorohydrate—it's less likely than other aluminum salts to trigger an allergic reaction. If the problem persists, switch to a deodorant—especially a fragrance-free deodorant, since unscented products of any kind are less likely to irritate skin than scented ones.

One possible choice is baking soda, now found in several underarm products. It absorbs wetness and can act as a mild, natural deodorant when used alone under the arms after bathing, particularly in cooler weather when perspiration is minimal.

To further reduce the likelihood of irritation, wait at least an hour after shaving to apply an antiperspirant or deodorant. For example, you may decide to shave before bedtime and apply your underarm product in the morning.

EYEWEAR FOR WORK AND PLAY

Walk into any optical store or optician's office, eyewear prescription clutched in your hand. The first thing you'll probably notice is a display of row upon row of frames. You try on a few pairs and finally settle for one you think looks best on you. But is your choice really the most flattering? How can you tell?

Eyewear is an extension of your face. So the eyewear you choose should harmonize with *your* facial features—your eyes, your nose and the shape of your face.

To choose the style of eyewear that most flatters your face, consider the cosmetic features listed in "Tips for Choosing Eyewear," and "Framing Your Face."

Of course, your eyewear has to feel good as well as look good, and that's where an optician can be helpful. Whether frames fit comfortably depends on the fit of the bridge, the part that rests on your nose, says Ralph Drew, eyewear consultant and author of the book *Professional*

Ophthalmic Dispensing. It's the bridge, not the stems, of your glasses that supports the weight of your lenses. On the wrong nose, certain bridge designs can be very uncomfortable and even unattractive. If the bridge doesn't fit properly, for example, your frames can leave painful and unsightly red marks on your nose. If the bridge fails to hug your nose at the proper point, your glasses may repeatedly slip forward. The heavier your lenses and frames, the more likely they are to slip and therefore the more important it is that the bridge fit well.

No two noses are alike, so insist that the optician take considerable care choosing and fitting your bridge. Remember, too, that you don't have to settle for frames the optician has in stock. Designs can be ordered expecially for you, or an existing frame can be modified to suit you.

SUNGLASSES FOR HEALTH, NOT STEALTH

Strictly speaking, "shades" don't merely shade your eyes—they also can absorb invisible ultraviolet light. That kind of action is good, because ultraviolet light rays can inflame the tender cornea of your eyes in the same way they can burn unprotected skin. And—like sunscreen for skin—the amount of protection needed varies from one person to another. Blue-eyed blondes, for example, need darker sunglasses than brown-eyed brunettes.

Skiers who spend hours on the slopes without protective eyewear are prone to eye pain and temporary loss of vision, known as actinic keratitis. But glare from reflected snow, sand or water can leave anyone's eyes tired and strained by the end of the day.

Brown-tinted lenses that filter out 70 percent or more of ultraviolet light are best for skiing, sailing and other sports that expose you to both direct and reflected light, especially in high altitudes or hot climates. Polarized lenses further reduce glare reflected from sand, snow or water because they're coated with a thin layer of special plastic that deflects any light rays approaching your line

Framing Your Face

If your face is wide, try wearing clear or light-colored frames that are high at the temples, with upswept lower rims. These make your face appear longer and slimmer. Avoid square or rectangular frames.

If your face is long, fairly dark, solid-color frames with low and curved or rounded temple pieces shorten your face. Avoid upswept lower rims.

If your face is triangular, with a small or pointed chin, use slender, light-colored, round frames with flush temple pieces to deemphasize your upper face. Avoid heavy, dark, square frames.

If your face is pear shaped—wider at your jaw than at your temples—wear fairly large, heavy, dark-colored, oval frames. These will emphasize your eyes and temples. Avoid square or rectangular frames.

If your face is very round, with small features, use slender or rimless frames to deemphasize roundness. Avoid frames that are either very small or very large.

If your face is oval you can probably wear any shape frame, including squares.

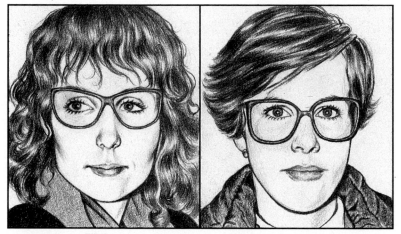

Wide   Long

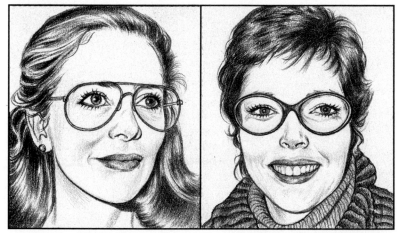

Triangular   Pear-shaped

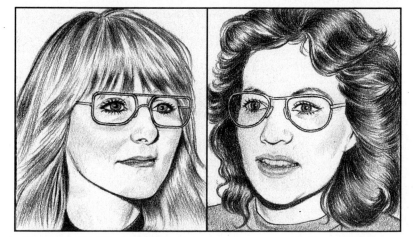

Very round with small features   Oval

of sight at a 90-degree angle.

Neutrally tinted lenses are the best choice for driving. Red, pink, rose or amber tints can fool you into seeing colors that don't really exist. For instance, a green light can look brown.

Not all sunglasses absorb ultra-violet rays adequately or polarize light. To be sure your sunglasses give you the protection you need, buy quality lenses from manufacturers who also supply prescription eyewear. These quality lenses are found at optical outlets, rather than at a carousel at the corner drugstore.

A Lifetime of Beauty

At each stage of life, certain changes occur that can alter your appearance. Luckily, many of the changes that accompany aging can be minimized, if you know what to do when. Women as young as 25, for example, need to be vigilant about exercise and calcium intake to protect themselves against the thinning bones and stooped posture of osteoporosis that often follows menopause. However, if you've already reached menopause, regular exercise and extra calcium can stop bone loss in its tracks and possibly even rebuild lost bone.

This chart presents tips for making the most of your beauty at every stage of life. You'll want to read over the entire plan to learn how to adopt lifelong beauty practices.

TEENS

Skin Care	Makeup	Hair Care	Exercise and Figure Control	Nutrition
Don't smoke cigarettes. Smoking eventually causes wrinkles and speeds up bone loss. If your face is oily, wash it twice a day. Use noncomedogenic, hypoallergenic cosmetics.	Use makeup sparingly, in light shades, to allow your fresh skin tones to show through and to prevent cosmetic-induced acne. Use water-based cosmetics if your skin is oily. Remove your makeup before going to sleep at night, and make it a lifelong habit.	Avoid tight pony tails, braids or other styles that can permanently pull out hair. Don't overdry your hair. Never brush when wet.	To control weight, exercise and eat moderate amounts of fish, poultry, vegetables and whole grains. Avoid crash diets, which deprive skin, hair and nails of protein and vitamins needed to look your best.	Eat liver and other high-iron foods or take iron supplements to make up for iron lost during menstruation. Avoid food binges or crash dieting.

20s

Skin Care	Makeup	Hair Care	Exercise and Figure Control	Nutrition
Your skin's in peak condition—make every effort to keep it that way. Protect yourself from the sun to prevent wrinkles and age spots. Pay special attention to your face, neck and hands—the most exposed yet delicate and vulnerable areas. Make it a habit to wear latex or cotton gloves for household chores and hobbies.	Experiment to find the makeup style that most flatters your face. You can carry off almost any look with flair.	Condition your hair regularly with a product formulated for your hair type (dry, oily or normal). Be careful not to over-condition, either by conditioning too often or with too rich a conditioner. Include hats in your work and play wardrobes to protect your hair from the drying effects of sun, wind or chill.	If you haven't played sports since high school or college, build exercise into your routine now. Consider participating in aerobics, dancercise, racquetball or other all-weather activities.	Use alcohol and caffeine sparingly, to avoid dry skin due to dehydration and stooped posture due to calcium losses. If you take birth control pills or suffer premenstrual syndrome, be sure to get enough vitamin B_6 from brown rice, salmon, liver, bananas, broccoli and sunflower seeds (or supplements) to counter depression or mood changes. Pay close attention to intake of protein and vitamins and minerals if you become pregnant.

30s

Skin Care	Makeup	Hair Care	Exercise and Figure Control	Nutrition
Always wear wrap-around dark glasses outdoors in bright light to prevent squint lines, crow's feet and drooping eyelids. Learn yoga or a related relaxation technique to cope with stress. Smooth moisturizing lotion over your feet every night to prevent callus buildup, especially if you walk much or play sports. Exercise to keep your skin from thinning out and losing elasticity.	At the first sign of a rash or blemishes, stop using makeup and investigate the cause. Use restrained, conservative makeup on the job, more elaborate makeup for leisure and evening hours.	Be sure your hairstyle is up-to-date and suits your face, job or lifestyle. The way you wore your hair when you were in your 20s may no longer be practical or flattering.	Do 25 bent-knee sit-ups a day to strengthen your back and flatten your stomach. Walk, cycle, dance, jump rope or do other exercises that work your calf muscles and pump blood through your legs to prevent varicose veins, counter stress and control weight. Weigh yourself once a week. Check any weight gain promptly by dieting.	Drink milk, eat low-fat dairy products and take a calcium supplement to prevent bone loss due to osteoporosis later. (Thin, petite women are most susceptible and need to pay special attention to dietary calcium.) Use butter and other animal fats sparingly. Eat strawberries, peppers and other foods high in vitamin C to fight off gum disease and tooth loss. High-fiber foods may also help to stave off varicose veins.

40s

Skin Care	Makeup	Hair Care	Exercise and Figure Control	Nutrition
Wash your face with a gentle, nondrying, easily rinsed soap or cleanser. Buff your face gently to speed up cell renewal. Always use a moisturizer to counteract dryness.	Always use a foundation makeup that contains a sunscreen. Use an undereye cover cream or concealer, if necessary. Avoid frosted or metallic shades of eye shadow if you have puffy or crepey eyelids. Use a lip base or lip pencil to anchor lip color and prevent lip color from feathering or bleeding beyond lip borders.	Frequent cuts can keep your hair looking its best at all times. If you decide to color your hair, make a hair coloring plan and stick to it. Figure out how often you'll need to color to keep roots covered and tint looking fresh all over.	If you've never exercised until now, get your doctor's go-ahead and pick an activity you think you might like, such as swimming or cycling. Go at it with moderate vigor. Lift hand weights to prevent upper arm flab.	Be sure to eat a lot of yellow fruit and vegetables—cantaloupe, sweet potatoes, squash and carrots—for their vitamin A, which is required for growth of new skin cells. If you're cutting calories, consider taking a multivitamin/mineral tablet.

50s

Skin Care	Makeup	Hair Care	Exercise and Figure Control	Nutrition
To prevent wrinkling around your neck, apply a rich moisturizing cream to your skin before going to sleep at night and apply a moisturizer with sunscreen whenever you're out in the sun. Protect fragile skin on your hands by *always* using a hand cream, preferably one with a sunscreen. Wear gloves. Wash with lukewarm water and mild soap. Soak nails in water for a few minutes before a manicure, to prevent brittleness.	Wear matte-finish foundation for moister-looking skin. Don't overapply makeup or you'll exaggerate lines and wrinkles. Avoid bright or frosted eye shadow if your lids are puffy or crepey. Wear muted, not red-blue, lipstick.	If your hair is gray, consider a short haircut, to flatter your face and maximize volume. If your hair seems wispy and thin, a perm and a conditioner for fine, limp hair can add body. If you have superfluous facial hair, decide on a method of temporary or permanent hair removal that suits you best.	To stimulate circulation in your legs, walk briskly 3 times a week. Swimming is great for arthritic knees and hips. Exercise in general can help skin to look plump and stay smooth. Exercise can also tone your stomach, strengthen bones, straighten posture and maintain high energy levels.	Be sure you're getting 1,200 milligrams of calcium a day from food or supplements. Spend some time outdoors every week to soak up enough vitamin D from sunshine to help keep bones strong. Before undergoing cosmetic surgery, take small amounts of vitamin E and zinc for a few weeks to speed healing.

Source Notes

Chapter 5

Page 25

"Skin-Saving Tips for the Sports Enthusiast" prepared with the assistance of Rodney Blasler, M.D., sportsmedicine dermatologist from the University of Nebraska.

Page 27

"An Answer to Acne: A Low-Iodine Diet" adapted from *Dr. Fulton's Step-by-Step Program for Clearing Acne* by James E. Fulton, Jr., M.D., Ph.D., and Elizabeth Black (New York: Harper & Row, 1983).

Photography Credits

Cover: Margaret Skrovanek
Staff Photographers—
Angelo M. Caggiano: pp. 30-31; 112-113; 155. Carl Doney: pp. 6-7; 66-67; 102; 146-147; 152-153. T. L. Gettings: pp. viii-1; 33. John Hamel: p. 23. Mark Lenny: pp. 34-35; 44; 54-55; 108. Alison Miksch: pp. 10; 12; 24; 36-37; 122. Margaret Skrovanek: pp. 41; 45; 56-57; 69; 72-73; 96; 104-105; 114; 126-127; 132; 134; 135; 140-141; 154. Christie C. Tito: pp. 4; 5; 9; 14; 70-71; 76-77; 78; 82-83; 88-89; 93; 94; 100-101; 106-107; 118; 138-139; 143; 156-157. Sally Shenk Ullman: pp. 90-91; 116; 144-145.

Other Photographers—
John Knutila: pp. 20-21. Gunter Marx/Devaney Stock Photos: p. 3, right.

*Additional Photographs Courtesy of—*Frederic Lewis, Inc.: pp. 2; 3, left.

Photographic Styling Credits

Anne Hakanson: pp. 6-7; 66-67; 88-89. Renee R. Keith: pp. 72-73. Kyle Traylor: pp. 144-145.

Illustration Credits

Bascove: pp. 28-29; 68; 156-157; 159. Susan Blubaugh: pp. 20-21; 38; 149. Susan Gray: pp. 16; 22; 64; 79; 128; 130. Mary Anne Shea: pp. 26; 58-59; 61; 98-99; 119; 133; 136-137; 138-139. Wendy Wray: pp. 33; 41; 42-43; 77; 80-81; 120-121; 161.

Special Thanks to—
Barely Legal, Gardena, Calif.; Caswell-Massey, New York; J. H. Diamond Company, Lake Worth, Fla.; Donna Baumann Gottlieb, color consultant, Washington, D.C. (pp. 138-139); Mary Jane Co., North Hollywood, Calif.; Leroy R. Perry, D.C., International Sportsmedicine Institute, West Los Angeles, Calif.; (p. 130); Rockport, Marlboro, Mass.; Schneck Optical, Emmaus, Pa; Levi Strauss & Co., San Francisco, Calif.; Jean Marie Turioscy, makeup specialist, Jean Marie Boutique, Allentown, Pa.

Index

Rodale Press, Inc., publishes PREVENTION®, the better health magazine.
For information on how to order your subscription,
write to PREVENTION®, Emmaus, PA 18049.